By the Sea

Dedicated to my husband, Brian, whose love and support made this possible.

And to my parents, Lorraine and Harry, who fostered my love of nature.

An Hachette UK Company
www.hachette.co.uk

First published in Great Britain in 2019 by Aster, a division of Octopus Publishing Group Ltd, Carmelite House, 50 Victoria Embankment, London EC4Y 0DZ
www.octopusbooks.co.uk

Distributed in the US by Hachette Book Group, 1290 Avenue of the Americas, 4th and 5th Floors, New York, NY 10104

Distributed in Canada by Canadian Manda Group, 664 Annette St, Toronto, Ontario, Canada M6S 2C8

ISBN 978-1-78325-294-7

A CIP catalogue record for this book is available from the British Library.

Printed and bound in Europe.

10 9 8 7 6 5 4 3 2 1

Consultant Publisher Kate Adams
Senior Editor Leanne Bryan
Designer Jack Storey
Contributing Editor Jo Smith
Illustrator Grace Helmer
Cover Artwork Jenny Mc Connell Design, www.jennymcconnelldesign.com
Picture Research Manager Giulia Hetherington
Picture Library Manager Jennifer Veall
Production Manager Caroline Alberti

By the Sea

The therapeutic benefits of being in, on and by the water

Dr Deborah Cracknell

aster

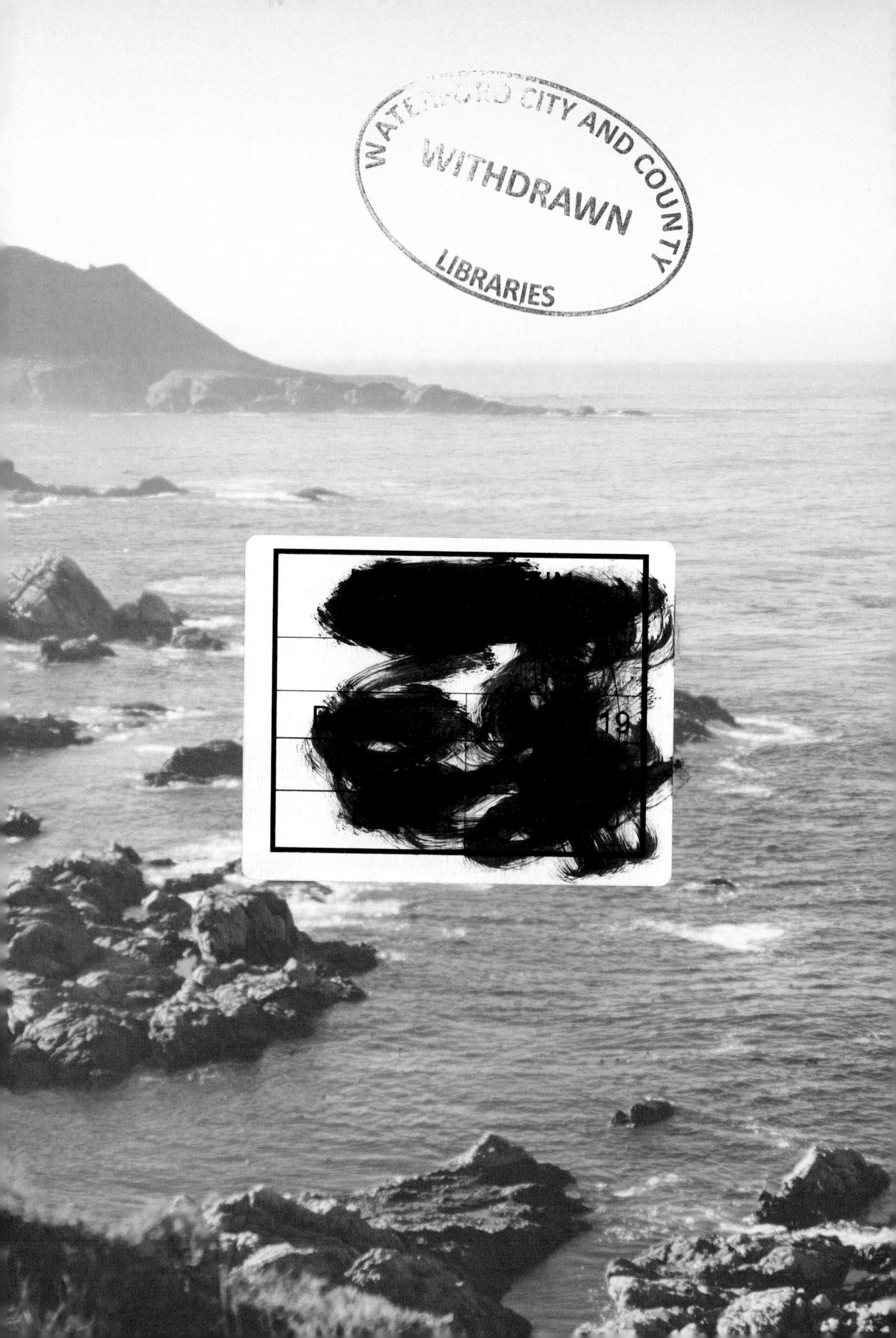

[redacted]

Contents

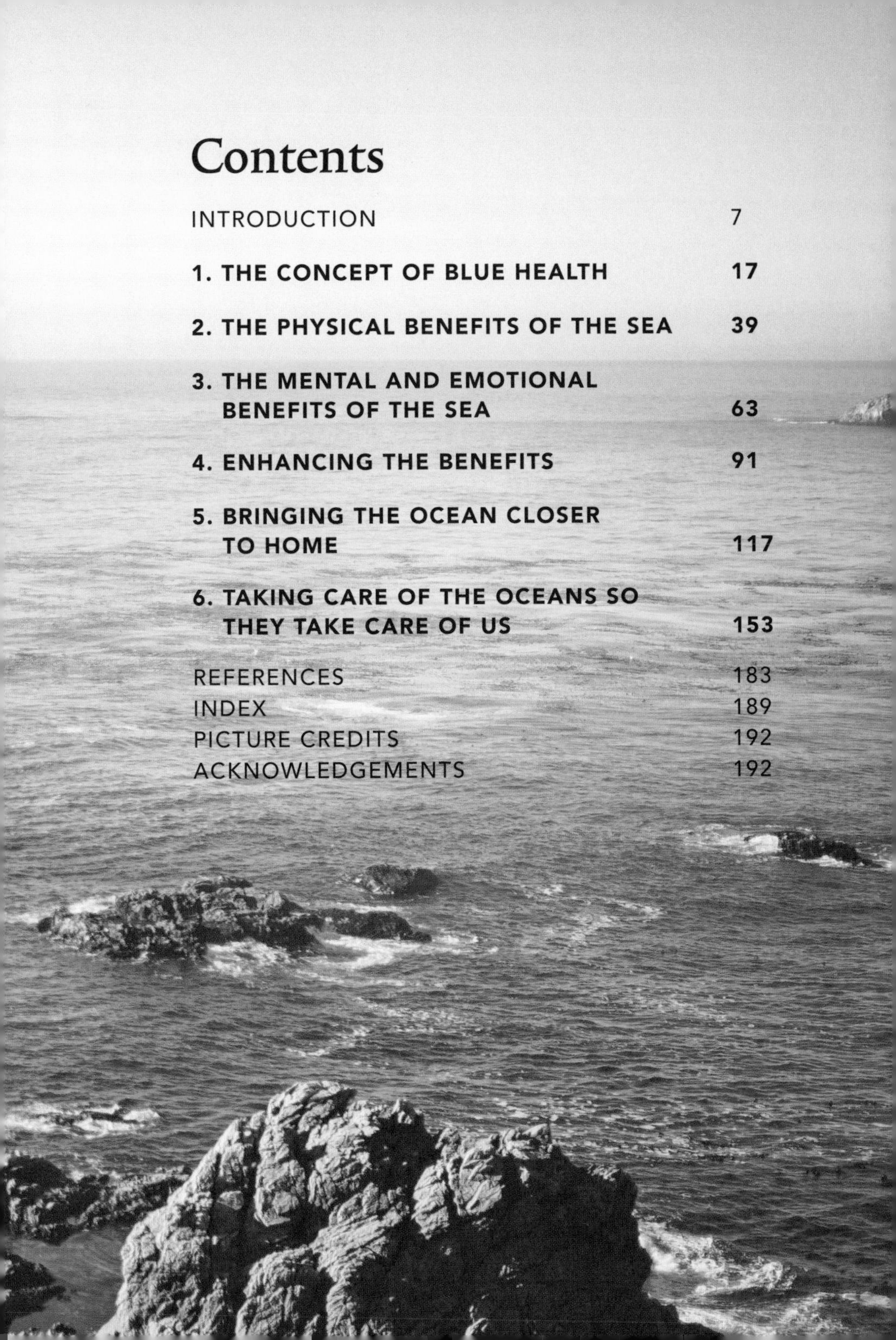

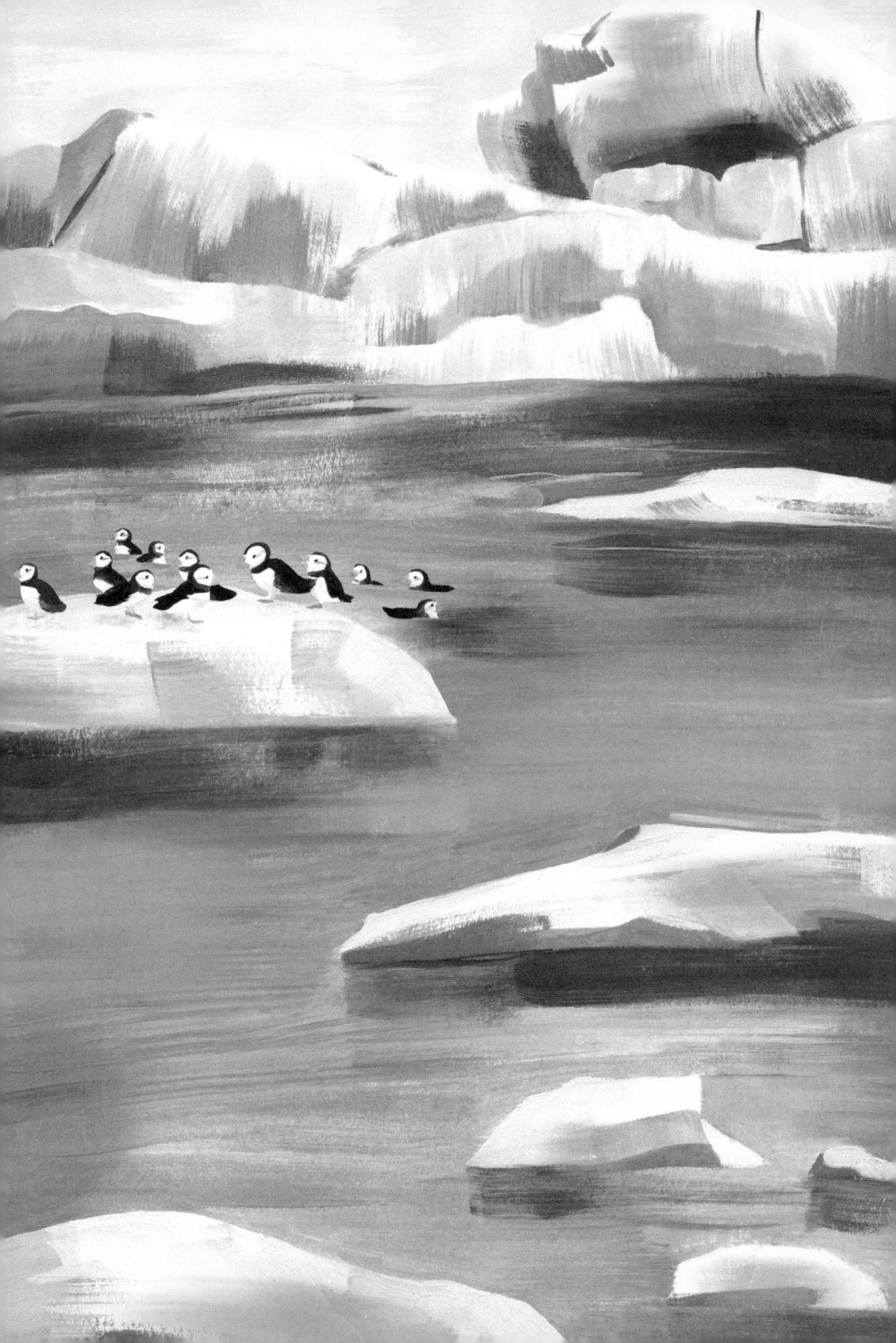

INTRODUCTION

"The sea, once it casts its spell, holds one in its net of wonder forever."

— Jacques Cousteau

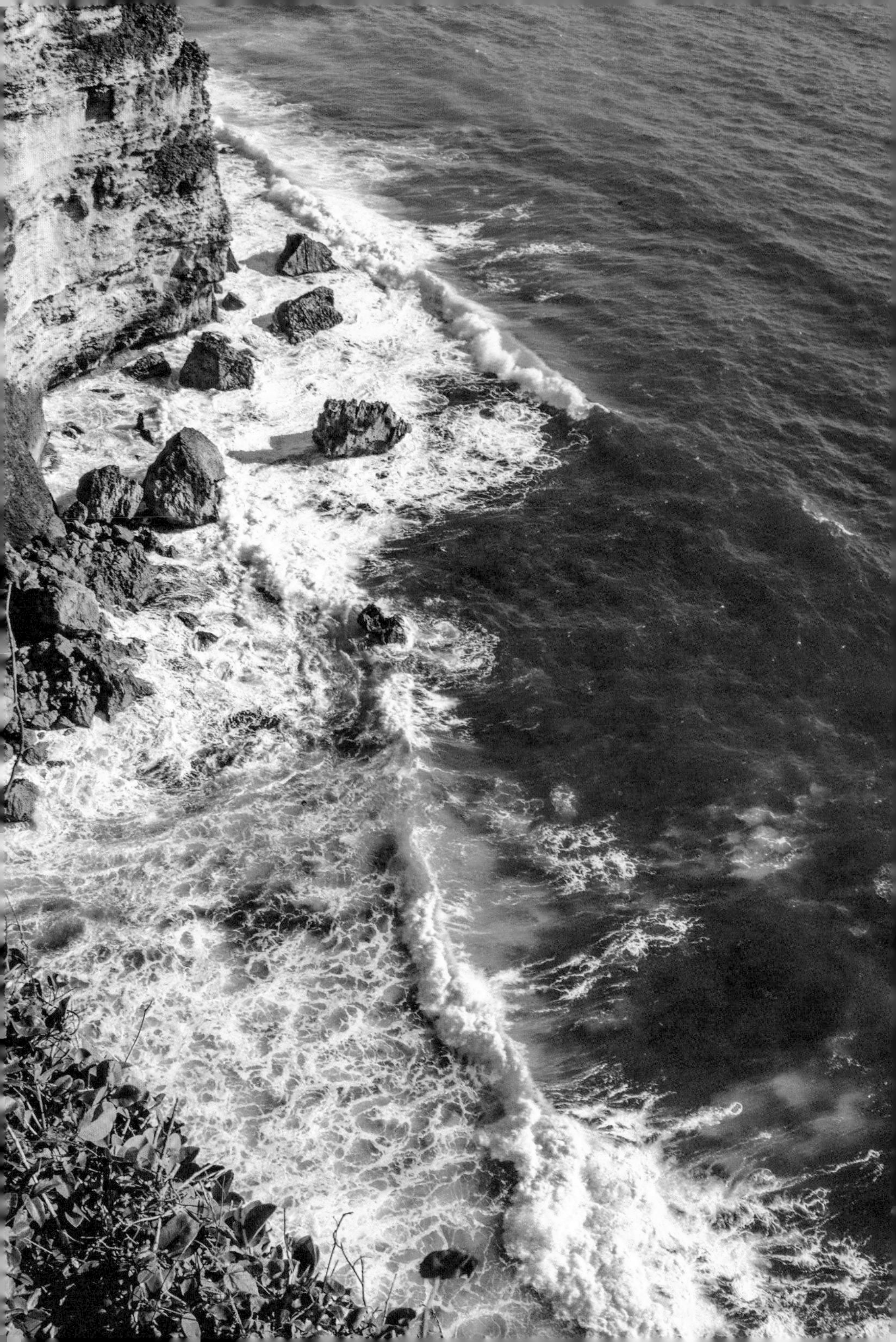

When you catch that first glimpse of blue as you are approaching the sea, it can make you smile, or take a slightly deeper breath, or want to quicken your pace in the anticipation of breathing in the ocean air and feeling the sun and wind on your face. It never ceases to be a moment of awe as you think – or even say out loud – "I can see the sea!".

The great vastness of the oceans, which cover 71 per cent of the earth's surface, contain 97 per cent of the earth's water and constitute 99 per cent of the earth's living space,[1] are a source of fascination, intrigue, beauty and unparalleled life.

Ancient cities have been engulfed by oceans and, beneath the surface, there are mountain ranges, valleys and canyons just as there are on dry land. More than 3.5 billion people rely on the oceans for their primary source of food, while 10 per cent of the world's population relies on the oceans for their livelihood. In fact, the very existence of humankind and all the creatures on the planet relies on the oceans to capture carbon, produce oxygen and make fresh water available for food production.

Around 40 per cent of the world's population lives within about 60 miles (1km) of the coast,[2] and 23 of the world's 30 largest cities are located on the coast.[3] The oceans are critical to our health and wellbeing in so many ways: the oceans provide a vital source of food; support individuals' livelihoods and large-scale commerce; provide transportation routes; supply valuable new medicines; regulate the climate; present opportunities for recreation and leisure; and are a source of beauty and inspiration.[4] Added to this, well over half of the oxygen in the atmosphere originates from marine plants, so every person on the planet benefits from, and is affected by, the oceans.

It would be impossible to chart the full history of our relationship with the sea, as we evolved from the first creatures to emerge on dry land to the complex creatures we are today. The oceans have been a primary source of nourishment – then exploration, trade and travel – since the beginning of human history. In his book *On the Ocean*, in which he explores the relationship between humans and the seas, Sir Barry Cunliffe points out that there is no history without the oceans – they are there at every turn, demanding invention and courage as early peoples developed the first crafts to cross them, feeding the innate human desire to explore and discover, at the same time inviting, wild and potentially dangerous.

"Is not the core of nature in the heart of man?"
—Johann Wolfgang von Goethe

In Homer's *Odyssey* the sea represents danger and wildness, and the weakness of man in contrast to the power of the Gods. Through the ages, the way in which philosophers have viewed the relationship between man and nature has been a journey in itself, from one of fear, to one of conquering, followed by a sense of stewardship and even kinship.

It is this sense of kinship – that our ability to thrive as a species is somehow linked to our environment – that scientists are now investigating. Those of us lucky enough to spend time in nature have a sense that it is good for us, that we are influenced by our surroundings both physically and emotionally. There is growing scientific interest in the benefits that nature can provide, especially the part that it may play as a form of preventative medicine through the positive effects on physical fitness and mental health and wellbeing. And how, if we look after the oceans, they will in turn look after us.

"To unpathed waters, undreamed shores..."
—William Shakespeare

MY BACKGROUND

I thought I'd let you know a little about myself and how I came to be researching the health and wellbeing benefits of being by the sea. I was born in 1966 in Plymouth, a city on the south-west coast of England. When recalling my childhood, I realize that my earliest and fondest memories are those connected with nature, especially those involving the sea. The house where I grew up had a big back garden full of flowers, bushes and wildlife. A large section of the garden was devoted to growing vegetables, and I spent many hours helping my father and learning all about the plants and animals that lived there.

I spent as much time as possible involved with the natural environment, invariably in or around water – learning to swim and playing in the sea, navigating slippery rocks in rivers and searching for tadpoles in ponds. My favourite times, however, were spent exploring rockpools at the beach. While I was fascinated to watch and learn all about the different creatures in this strange watery world, my father had an additional reason for ensuring that I was able to correctly identify the different species on the rocky shore – he was very partial to collecting, cooking and eating winkles.

Through my father's love of foraging and my mother's fondness for flowers, I became in tune with the seasons. I enjoyed watching the succession of flowers and plants throughout winter and spring – peeping snowdrops, nodding daffodils, clusters of primroses and stunning carpets of woodland bluebells, followed by the heady scent of summer honeysuckle. Autumn brought foraging opportunities as we searched for fallen sweet chestnuts among the red and golden leaves. And although present year round, spotting the first robin of winter always seemed to herald the exciting approach of Christmas – and the New Year, when the annual cycle of nature would begin again.

I was fortunate enough to live in a time when children were allowed to spend all day with their friends, occasionally popping home for a midday snack but, more often than not, simply being out and about all day, only returning home for tea. Many summer holidays were spent making dens in woods, riding bikes, paddling in streams, lazing around in meadows (usually searching for a four-leaf clover), and generally getting wet and muddy.

I did quite well at school – more through hard work and determination than any academic flair – and particularly enjoyed biology. I started my A levels at 16 but, lacking direction, I left school and went to work in a

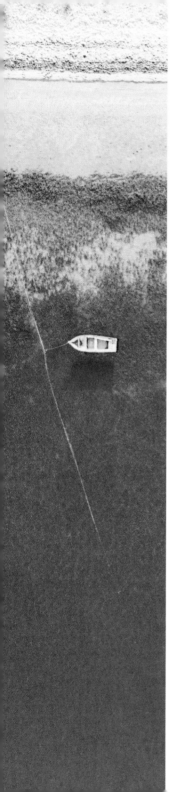

bank as a stop gap, while I decided what I wanted to do with my life. Although I very quickly realized that working in the financial services industry was not for me, earning my own money did enable me to enjoy watersports and holidays by the sea.

My temporary stop gap drifted on for almost 12 years. During this time, however, I'd always retained my love of the sea and biology, even trying to find a marine biology evening class in the hope that this be a way to help change my career direction. Alas, no such course was available, and I was convinced that the financial services industry was my path for life until a chance conversation opened my eyes to another possibility: go to university and start again.

I started a science foundation course at the University of Plymouth before starting my BSc. (Hons) in Marine Biology with Microbiology, in 1995. As a mature student I felt the need to ensure that I took as many opportunities as I could to get ahead, and I spent each summer either volunteering at the University's aquarium facility or in their fish nutrition laboratory. During this period, I also learned to scuba dive and undertook several recreational diving courses. On the final day of one particular course, just as we surfaced after our final dive, the boat skipper excitedly informed us that a large basking shark was in the area. We quickly ditched our diving gear and disappeared back over the side of the boat with our masks and snorkels, just in time to see the basking shark right in front of us, mouth agape, feeding on the plankton. It was a magical experience and one that will stay with me forever.

I graduated three years later and decided to enhance my diving qualifications by enrolling on a four-week commercial diving course. It was then that the most serendipitous thing happened. A large new marine aquarium had opened up in Plymouth just a few months earlier and I had wandered around the aquarium exhibits on its public opening day, desperately wishing that

I could somehow join the team of biologist/divers that worked there. While I was sitting apprehensively in the dive centre waiting for the other participants on the course to turn up, another person joined me. We exchanged pleasantries and he asked me why I was doing the diving course. I chatted away – relieved of something to take my mind off the impending course – and explained that I'd just finished my degree and was hoping to get a marine biology job, preferably one that involved diving. I told him about a new aquarium that had just opened, and how wonderful it would be to work there and dive in the tanks. I suddenly then remembered that I hadn't asked him what he did. "Oh", he laughed, "I'm Head of Diving at the aquarium". What a coincidence!

As two marine biologists on the dive course, we got on well, and I started volunteering at the National Marine Aquarium in Plymouth shortly after the course finished. I was then fortunate to secure a full-time position as a biologist/diver two months later and spent the next 19 years working at the aquarium. During this time, I had a variety of roles: looking after the animals and diving in the exhibit tanks; improving sustainability as environmental manager; and running a 10-year monitoring programme on an artificial reef on a decommissioned Royal Navy frigate, HMS *Scylla*. This final role was the start of a more active involvement with research and, before long, I was helping to develop and coordinate the aquarium's research and conservation activities.

During this time, my focus shifted from mainly animal-based studies to more people-based research, as I was introduced to the subject of Oceans and Human Health. This fascinating topic not only encompasses the various ways in which the oceans can negatively impact human health, often as a result of human activity (such as bathing in polluted seas), but also the positive effects the seas and oceans can have on our health and wellbeing.

I began a part-time PhD in 2010. As I'd spent many years observing how relaxing visitors found the aquarium exhibits, it seemed logical that my PhD focused on the health and wellbeing benefits of watching marine life in aquariums. I spent the next six years researching the effects of different marine species on psychological and/or physiological health and wellbeing. I have presented my findings at national and international conferences, published a number of scientific journal articles and given several interviews for radio programmes, newspapers and other periodicals – all things I could never have imagined doing when younger!

In 2017, the aquarium found itself no longer able to support a research programme, so my career has taken another twist, providing opportunities to develop work and research ideas with new individuals and organizations – as well the valuable chance to write this book. I am delighted to have been given this opportunity, which I see as an important way to communicate scientific research to a wider audience, beyond the purely academic world. I hope this book will provide useful tips on how we can better experience the sea, so that our greater connection to the oceans – and awareness of the threats they face – further inspire us to take care of this precious environment. I am, in many ways, starting a new chapter and I hope you enjoy reading this book as much as I have enjoyed writing it.

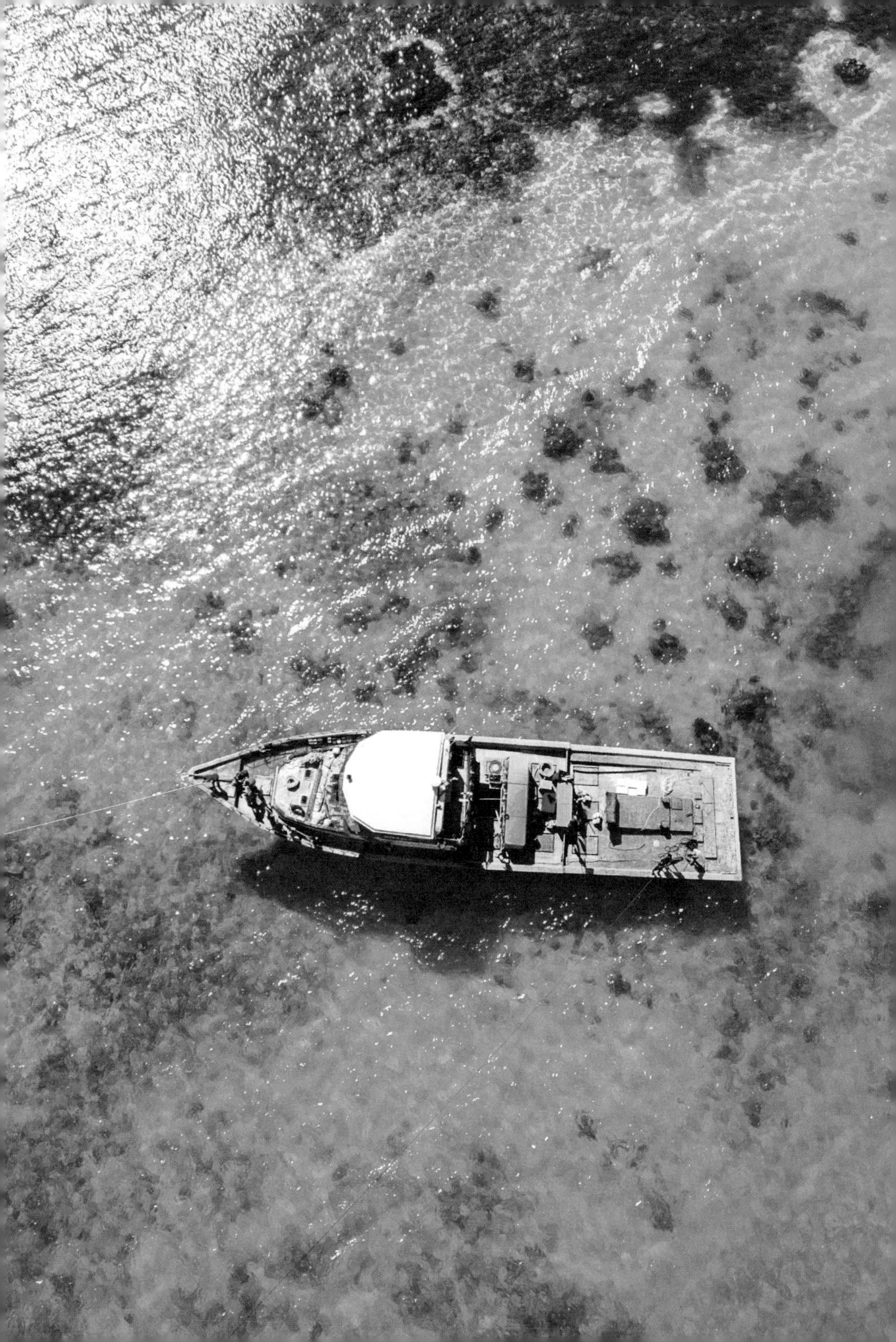

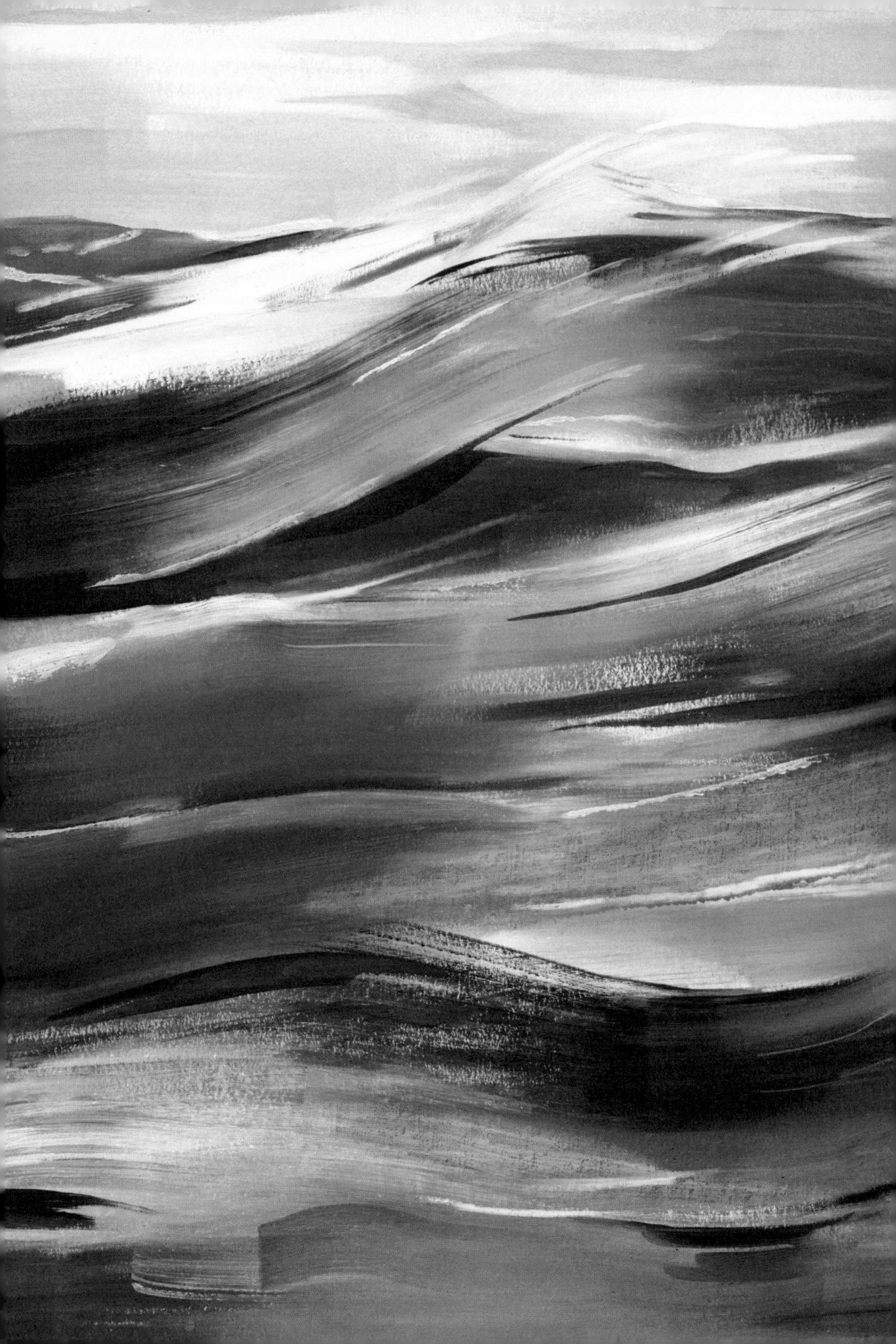

CHAPTER 1

The Concept of Blue Health

"Why do we love the sea?
It is because it has some
potent power to make
us think things we
like to think."

— Robert Henri

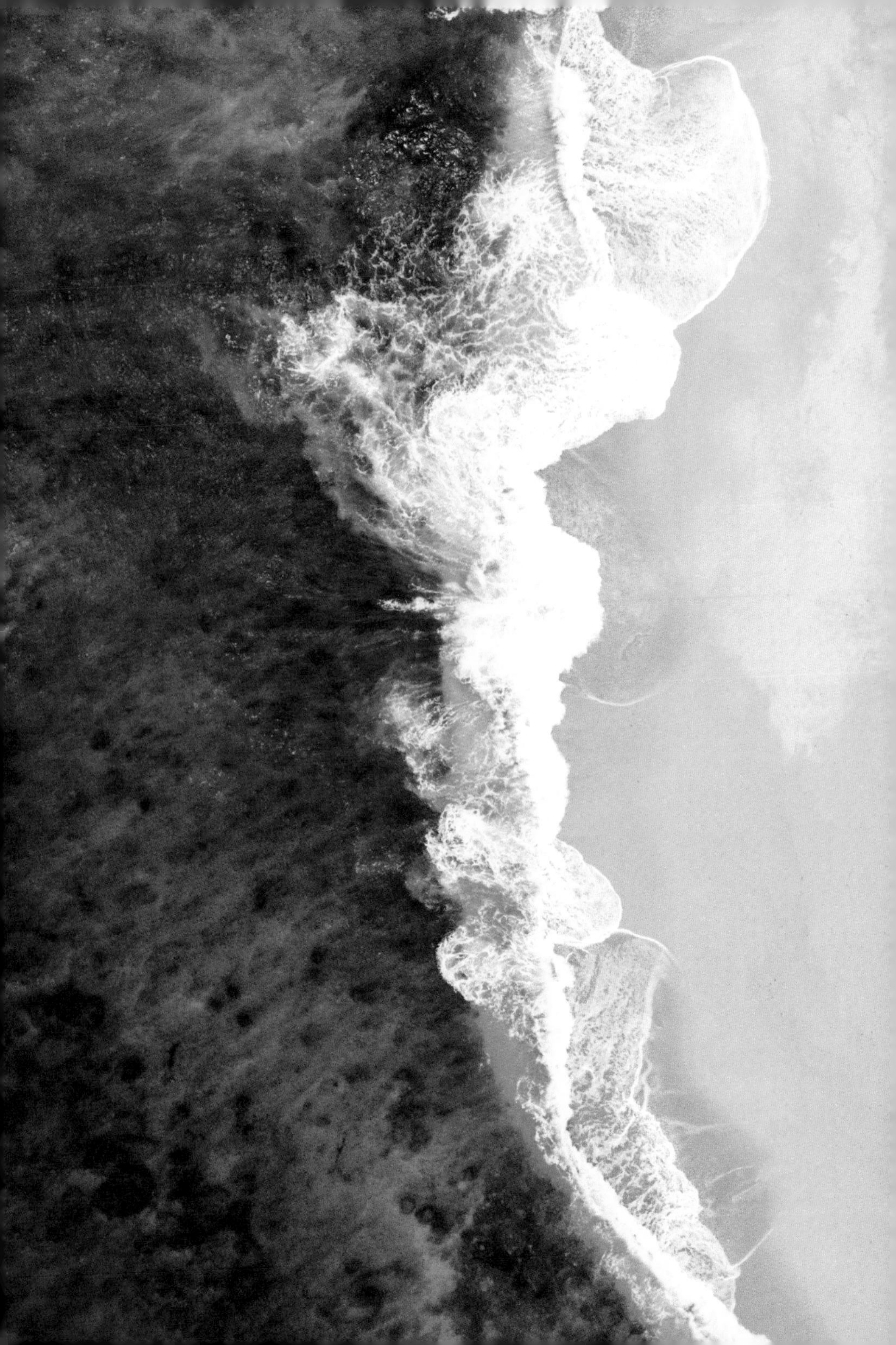

It is generally accepted that the first signs of life on our planet were found in the oceans, billions of years ago.[5] Much later – around 450 million years ago – the first animal footprints appeared on land. Evolution continued, and a fantastic array of organisms developed over time to populate land, air and sea. Eventually *Homo sapiens*, the species to which modern humans belong, evolved around 300,000 years ago.

Humans have had a long relationship with the sea, so it's not surprising that our inquisitive nature has encouraged us to explore the myriad connections we have with it. It is a source of food, medicine, pleasure and leisure. And one of the reasons that we seek a better understanding of our relationship with the sea is the increasing realization that it can have a whole host of beneficial effects on our health, wellbeing and quality of life.

We can gain so many different physical and mental health benefits from the oceans: walking along the coast or swimming in the sea contributes to our physical activity needs; visiting the beach with family and friends fosters valuable social interaction; spending time in natural environments promotes positive relationships with nature; watching and listening to the ocean relaxes us and calms our busy minds; consuming seafood provides an important source of protein and nutrients; and marine-sourced pharmaceuticals help treat a wide variety of medical illnesses.[6,7] Some of these benefits are a result of direct contact with the sea, whereas others come by more indirect routes: all, however, can positively contribute to our physical and mental health and wellbeing.

WHAT DO WE MEAN BY "HEALTH" AND "WELLBEING"?

The World Health Organization (WHO) defines health as "a state of complete physical, mental and social wellbeing and not merely the absence of disease or infirmity."[8] It means that a person can realize his or her own abilities, cope with the stresses of everyday life, work productively and contribute to their community.[9, 10] A dictionary may simply define wellbeing as "the state of being comfortable, healthy or happy", but perhaps a better description would be closer to the WHO definition of health, suggesting that stable wellbeing occurs when people have the physical, mental and social resources they need to meet physical, mental and/or social challenges.[11] It is worth emphasizing here that, although I will focus on the physical (body) or mental (mind) health benefits of being in or near the sea, it is impossible to separate the two: there really is a connection between a healthy body and a healthy mind.

HOW MENTAL HEALTH AND STRESS AFFECT US

Stress, unemployment and overwork can have a huge impact on our wellbeing. The *Oxford Dictionary* defines stress as "a state of mental or emotional strain, or tension resulting from adverse or demanding circumstances". It can manifest in a variety of different ways, causing psychological, physiological and behavioural symptoms.

- Psychologically, a stressful situation may result in emotions such as anger, fear and sadness, feeling overwhelmed with life, becoming easily agitated or having low self-esteem.
- Physiological symptoms – such as low energy, headaches, stomach problems, muscle tension and pain – may be caused by the cardiovascular, skeletomuscular and neuroendocrine systems being mobilized to cope with the situation. Mobilizing the body to deal with these stressful situations uses up resources and energy, which can contribute to fatigue.
- Behaviourally, people try to avoid stressful situations, and may perform poorly on tasks, or rely on harmful substances such as excess alcohol or nicotine to cope.[12]

Although a small amount of stress may help our performance in some situations, long-term chronic stress associated with everyday life can lead to mental health disorders such as anxiety and depression, and other health problems such as raised blood pressure, and the increased risk of heart disease and strokes.[13]

Mental health disorders and the effects of stress are a serious concern for individuals, but they can also have a devastating impact on their family and friends. They also put a large burden on society as it struggles to cope with the financial demands of dealing with its citizens' health issues. In Great Britain alone, approximately 12.5 million work days were lost in 2016/2017 due to stress, anxiety or depression, at a cost of billions of pounds.[14,15] This is a global problem: worldwide more than 300 million people are living with depression and over 260 million people suffer with anxiety disorders.[16]

Although medication can help alleviate some mental ill health symptoms, it is costly and can have undesirable side effects. Furthermore, medication does not work for many individuals in the medium to long term. It's not surprising that the healthcare sector is increasingly exploring alternative treatments to complement the modern medical approach.

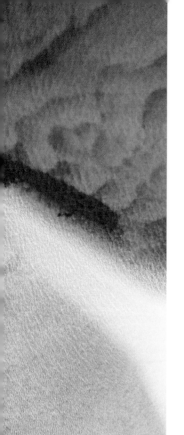

HOW NATURE CAN BENEFIT HEALTH AND WELLBEING

One alternative to medication is the use of natural environments as a "cure" for many of life's health and wellbeing problems.[17] Considering that many people intuitively respond to the stress and mental fatigue in their lives by seeking out natural environments in which they can relax and mentally take time out,[18] the idea that nature can provide a means of stress recovery and enhance wellbeing is worth investigating. Indeed, we have been using nature as "therapy" throughout history. But to some extent, in recent years, we have lost touch with the healing effects of nature because of the advances and applications of modern medicine.[19]

However, the efficiency and convenience of modern medicine is not the only reason that we are less aware of the health benefits that nature can bring; our changing world and "progressive" lifestyles are also having an effect. An increasing population is resulting in an expanding built environment – often at the expense of precious natural settings – and developments in digital technology, such as smart phones and tablets, provide us with almost limitless ways in which to occupy our free time. It is thought that today's children are particularly affected. Parental fear of "stranger danger" and busy roads, coupled with so much screen time, is resulting in children spending less time outdoors and in nature.

There has always been historical evidence of our connection to nature – through art and literature, for instance – yet most of the experimental research on its positive effect on our health and wellbeing has developed since the mid-20th century. This seems largely in response to the marked increase in physical and mental health disorders since this time and the need to find additional ways to address these problems.[20]

Restorative Environment Research

The idea that nature can provide a way to relieve stress and promote greater wellbeing has prompted research into "restoration" and "restorative environments". Restoration can be defined as "the process of renewing physical, psychological and social capabilities diminished in ongoing efforts to meet adaptive demands."[21] The effects of restoration could include physical and mental recovery from stressful situations, or the alleviation of mental fatigue.[12]

Although a restorative environment can be any place "urban" or "natural" that helps us recover from stress or chronic fatigue, more often than not these environments are natural settings. Natural environments tend to make people feel less stressed, make them more inclined to exercise, offer a place for positive social interaction and provide a better-quality environment with less air and water pollution, for example.[22]

So, in other words, we tend to find spending time in and around nature – and even simply viewing natural environments – improves our mood and helps us feel more relaxed and less stressed.

THE ROLE OF URBANIZATION

We know the pressures of everyday life can increase levels of stress and affect wellbeing, but it has also been proposed that the process of urbanization itself – the migration of people from rural to urban settings during the past 200 years – has contributed to an overall reduction in people's ability to cope with stress. We have evolved with nature over millions of years, but increasing urbanization means we spend less time exposed to nature's protective influences on our health.[20,23,24]

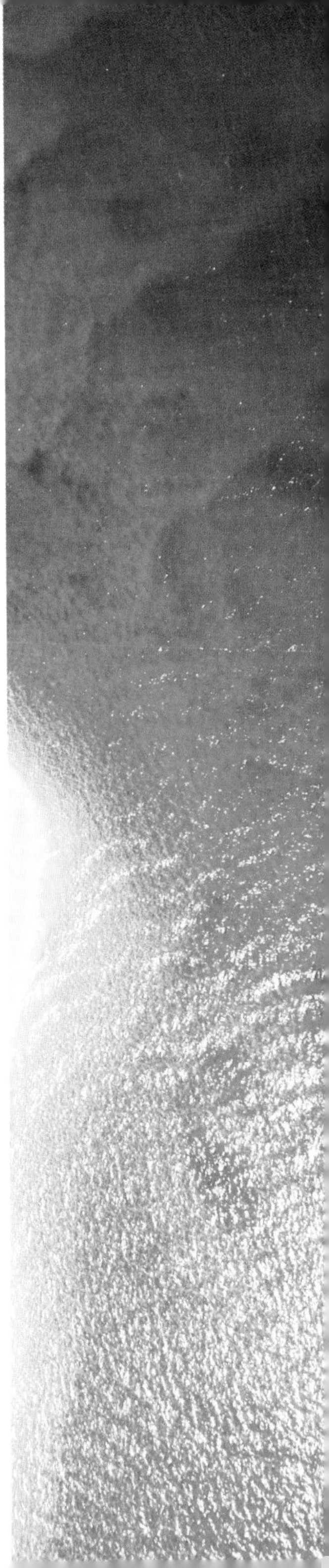

The importance of nature as an antidote to city living was highlighted by Frederick Law Olmsted, an influential landscape architect and planner in the United States. In the second half of the 19th century, increasing numbers of Americans were moving to cities and Olmsted wrote about his intuitive conviction that viewing nature could be an effective way of producing restoration and reducing the stresses associated with urban living. His beliefs about the restorative effects of nature influenced his public park designs in American cities and his work with the country's national parks.

Olmsted's views seem even more pertinent today. Since 1950, the urban population of the world has grown rapidly from 746 million to 3.9 billion. Currently, over half the world's population live in urban, rather than rural, areas: a rise of 24 per cent since 1950. Although levels of urbanization across the world differ, the United Nations anticipates that all regions will become more urbanized over the coming years, and the overall level will reach 66 per cent by 2030.

However, it is not just the number of people living in urban settings that gives cause for concern; it is the speed in which, from an evolutionary perspective, this has occurred. Millions of years of evolution in the natural world have resulted in humans developing automatic reactions to elements in nature that aid survival and wellbeing – for example, we tend to respond positively to water and vegetation, and negatively to snakes. In comparison, we have spent only a fraction of our history in built environments and, as such, have not yet evolved comparable responses to situations there.[25]

EARLY RESEARCH

While history has provided much anecdotal evidence of the health and wellbeing benefits of nature, it is only in the past few decades that there has been a surge in scientific studies.[22] One of the most well-known studies, by behavioural scientist Dr Roger S Ulrich, found that patients who had a view of trees from their hospital window stayed in hospital for a shorter time after surgery, took less pain medication, and tended to receive more favourable evaluations in nurses' notes during their recovery than those patients whose window faced a brick wall.[26] Since this early work, hundreds of studies have explored how people feel about and respond to

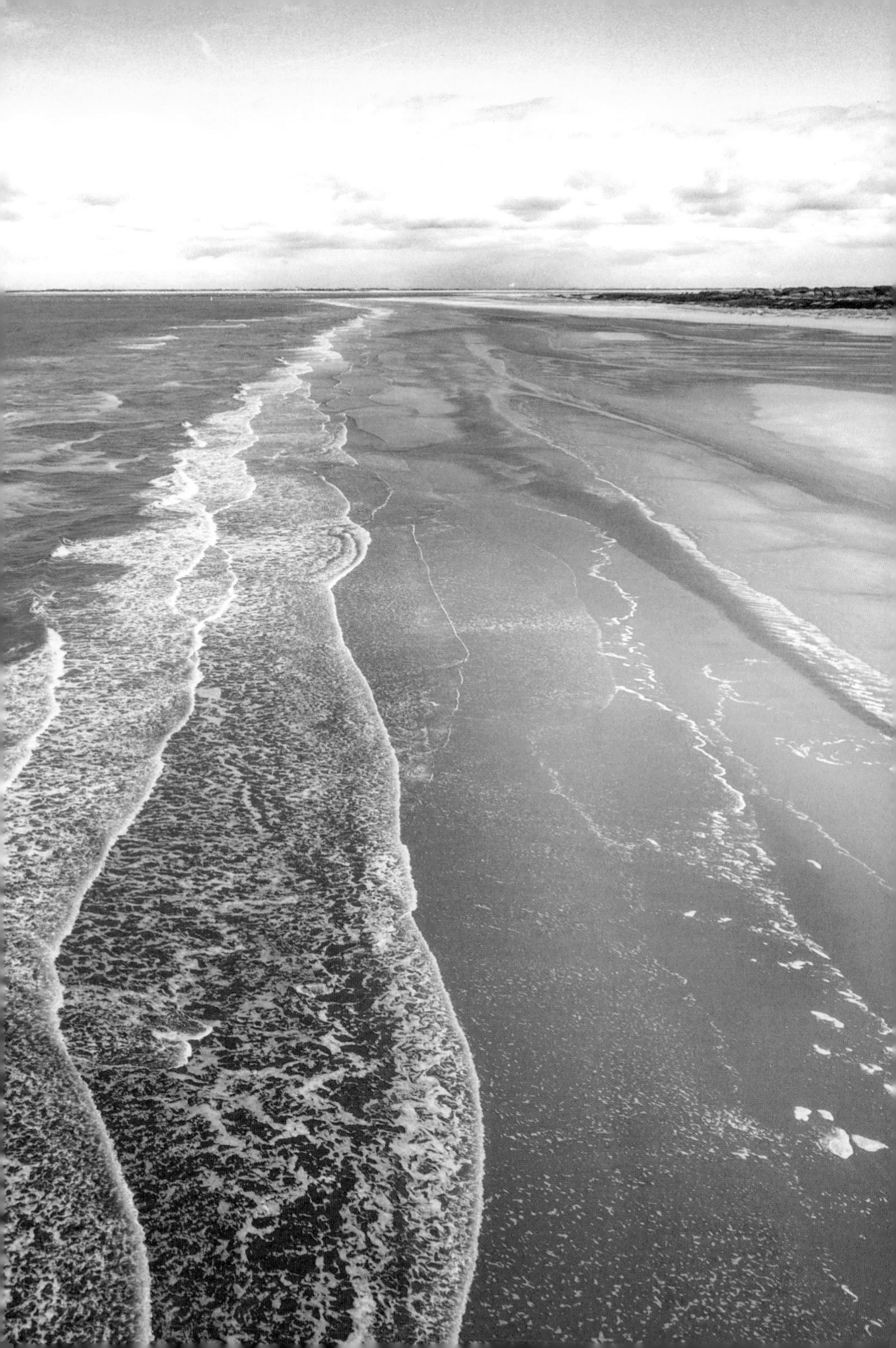

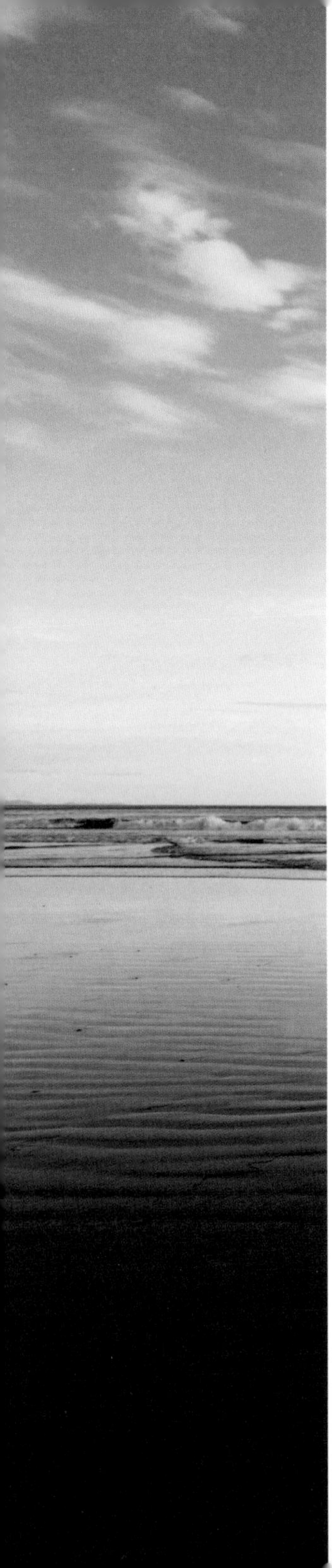

different environments. Many of these studies ask people how much they like certain landscapes, how pleasant and scenic they find them, and/or how psychologically and physiologically restorative they find them.[25,27]

Some studies have compared how people react to stress in natural and urban settings, comparing their psychological reactions (such as mood) and their physiological reactions (such as blood pressure).[28] However, as visiting and monitoring people's responses to many different places can be logistically difficult, much of this research uses simulations of landscapes – such as colour photographs and slides,[29,30] videos,[12,31,32] art[33,34] and virtual reality[35,36] – and takes place in research laboratories.

It is likely, however, that the real environment more fully engages our senses, resulting in a more powerful and immersive experience.[37–42]

Overall, there is now an extensive body of scientific evidence to show that people prefer environments that feature some natural elements, such as vegetation, flowers or water, and that these settings are beneficial for people's physical and mental health. They can improve wellbeing by increasing positive emotions and reducing stress and mental fatigue, particularly when compared with urban settings.[18,19,22,43,44]

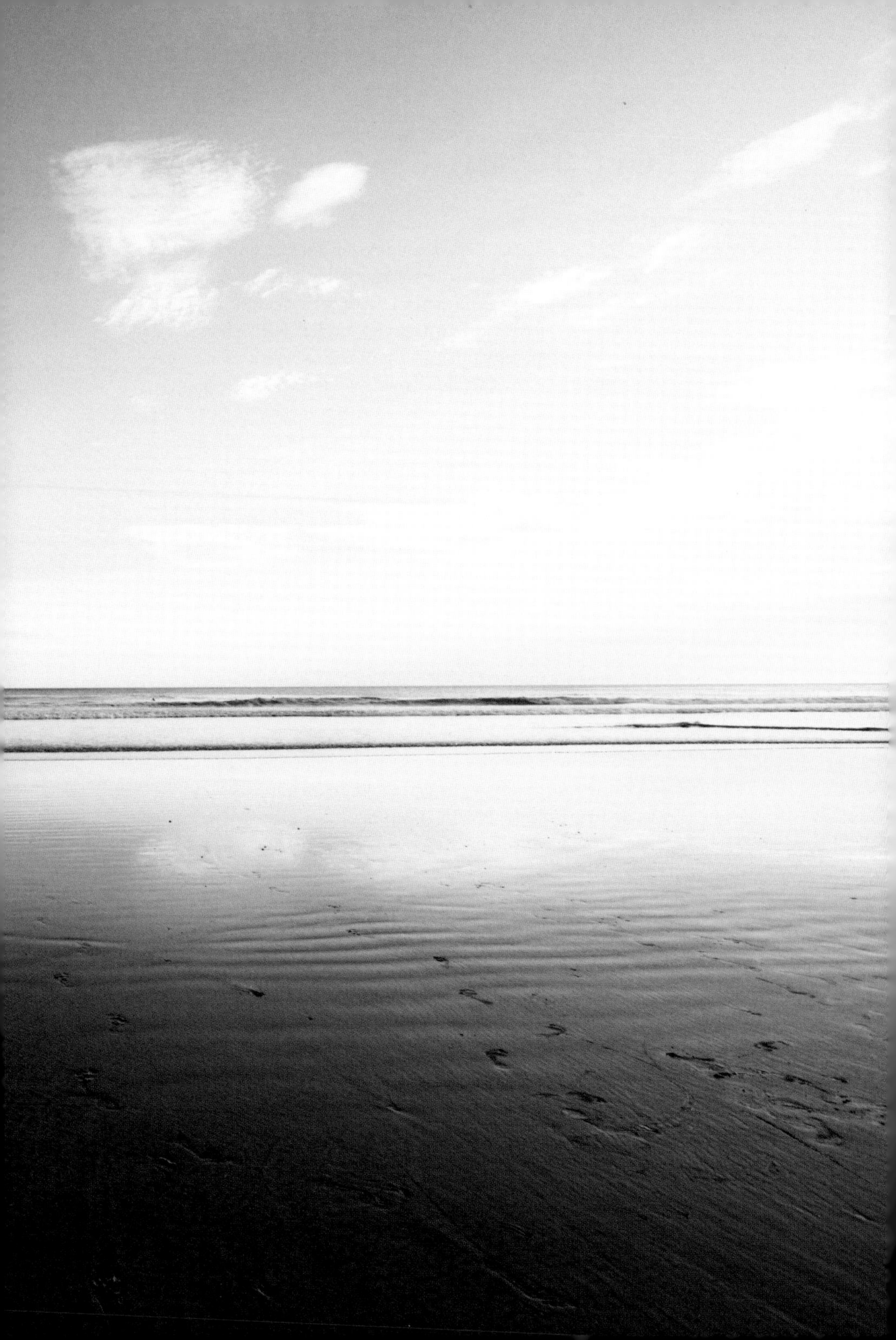

Our Love of "Blue"

Intriguingly, it is some of our daily behaviours that hint at our preference for blue spaces. We tend to prefer views that contain water to those that do not, and we are willing to pay more for such views: waterside properties are usually more expensive than comparable inland properties,[45] and hotel rooms with a sea view typically command the highest prices.[46] It is suggested that our willingness to pay more for these waterside views is because we believe that we derive some benefit from them.[47]

Water is a feature of landscapes that we find fascinating and aesthetically pleasing. We are drawn to water as it can evoke positive feelings such as relaxation and tranquillity.[25] Although we may feel and act upon this intuitively, this is also supported by scientific research. Studies have found that the natural settings that people especially like tend to contain water.[25, 27] These preferences are not confined to adults; young children show strong positive responses to water, and even infants and toddlers have been observed mouthing and licking shiny, glossy surfaces, such as mirrors, suggestive of glistening water.[48]

Furthermore, historical evidence and scientific studies suggest that responses to certain landscape features and configurations are remarkably similar across cultures.[25] For instance, people often express a preference for certain vegetation and tree canopy shapes that are typical of savannah-type landscapes. It is thought that pre-modern humans may have associated these landscapes with a good chance of finding food and water, so we are still drawn to them to this day.[12]

THE DEVELOPMENT OF "BLUE SPACE" RESEARCH

Noting the relative lack of research on the "restorative" potential of water, a team of researchers from the UK undertook a series of studies to investigate people's responses to aquatic environments. They found that the presence of water was a confounding factor in several studies comparing people's responses to natural and urban settings.[49] For example, in one study 39 out of 50 "nature" photographs contained water, whereas water did not feature in any "urban" photographs.[50] The researchers considered the lack of water in urban scenes a possible oversight considering that many towns and cities are located near water.

Although a small number of studies had specifically looked at aquatic environments,[51] overall there was a lot more work to be done.

To increase our understanding of people's reactions to aquatic environments, researchers compared responses to different scenes of green space, blue space and urban settings. The researchers used 120 photographs of natural and built environments with standardized proportions of "aquatic", "green" and "built" elements (for example, one-third green and two-thirds aquatic). Study participants were asked several questions, including how attractive they found the scenes, how the photograph made them feel (rated on a scale from "very sad" to "very happy") and how "restorative" they thought the environment would be.

As in previous studies, they found that ratings for the natural environments were more positive than those for the built environments. They noted, however, that both natural and built scenes that contained water were rated higher than those without water.[49] Research is continuing to explore the health and wellbeing effects of blue space, particularly coastal environments, adding to our knowledge of this fascinating subject (see pages 40–61).

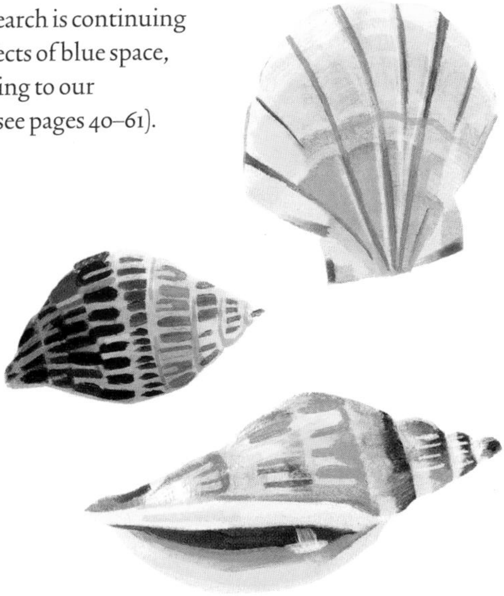

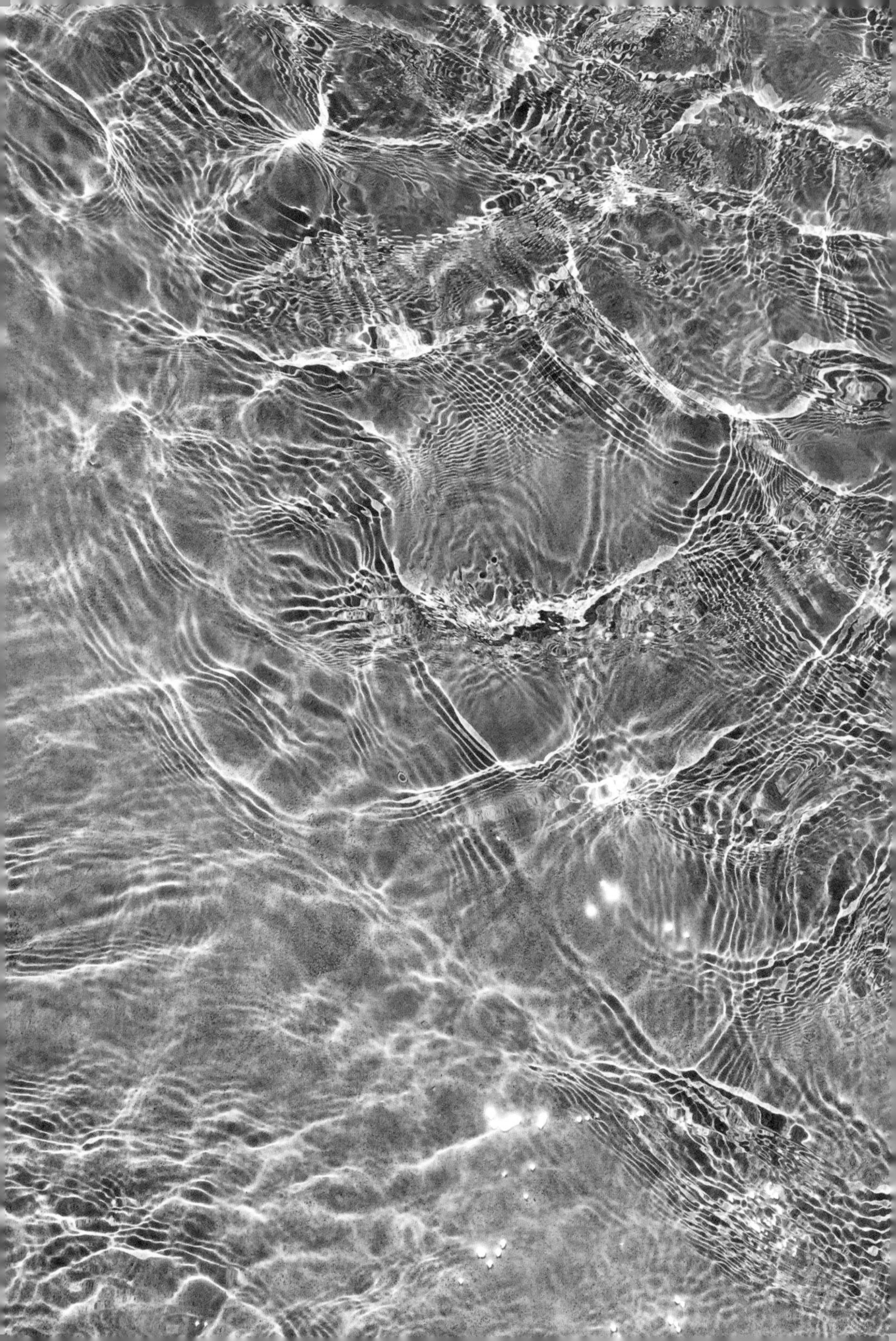

Why is Nature Restorative?

Several ideas have been proposed to explain why humans are drawn to, and may gain benefit from, natural environments. The three main approaches are the Biophilia Hypothesis, the Psychophysiological Stress Recovery Theory, and the Attention Restoration Theory.

BIOPHILIA HYPOTHESIS

The term "biophilia", meaning "love of life or living systems", was first used by psychoanalyst and social philosopher Erich Fromm in 1964,[52] but was later popularized by American biologist Edward O Wilson in his 1984 book *Biophilia*. Wilson's hypothesis proposes that throughout millions of years of evolution, humans have been inextricably linked to the natural environment and we are therefore genetically programmed to respond positively to elements of nature that support success and survival, and negatively to elements of nature that may harm us or hinder survival and wellbeing in some way. Furthermore, it is suggested that our inherent emotional connection to other living organisms is a basic human need, rather than just a cultural amenity or individual preference,[53,54] and if we don't maintain contact with natural systems and processes, our physical and mental wellbeing will suffer.[55]

PSYCHOPHYSIOLOGICAL STRESS RECOVERY THEORY (PSRT)

The PSRT (also known as the Stress Recovery Theory) was proposed by Dr Roger S Ulrich and also has an evolutionary basis. Ulrich suggests that, during natural selection, humans developed immediate and involuntary emotional and physiological responses to aspects of natural environments. For instance, when faced with an acutely stressful situation, the body's sympathetic nervous system triggers a fight-or-flight response, mobilizing the body for action by releasing hormones so that it can quickly deal with the evolving situation[12] – the heart beats faster, breathing increases, digestion decreases and the liver releases glucose for energy. This activation of bodily systems requires energy and is therefore physically exhausting.

This fight-or-flight response (also known as the acute stress response) evolved in humans and other mammals to enable them to respond

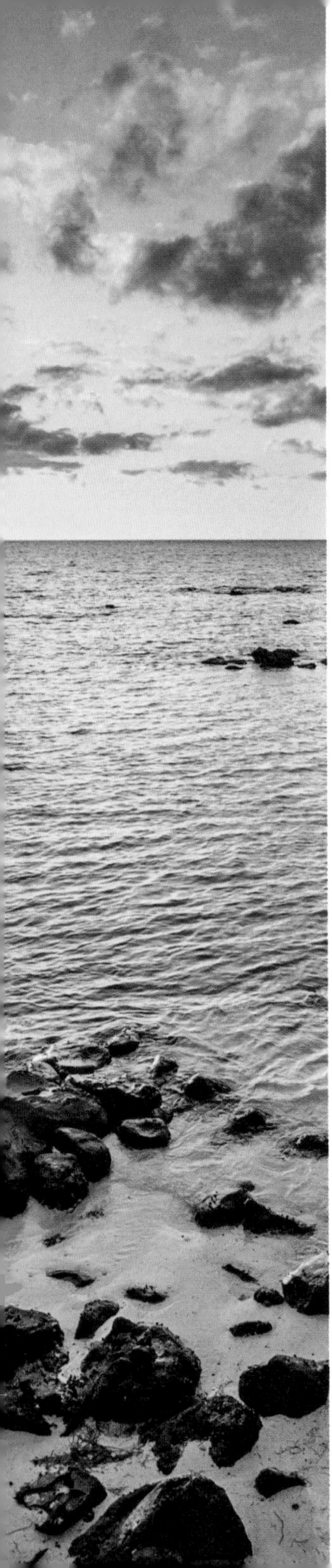

quickly to a harmful event, attack or a threat to survival. However, certain elements of modern-day living – the daily commute, pressure at work, family issues – can also activate the stress response. Eventually, recurring activation of the stress response can have a negative impact on physical and mental health; people suffering from chronic stress may experience high blood pressure, depression and anxiety, and poor sleep. Coping mechanisms may themselves be harmful: people may become reliant on alcohol or nicotine, or begin comfort eating to help them deal with their stress.

Just as the sympathetic nervous system prepares the body for immediate action, the parasympathetic nervous system restores the body to a state of calm. It stimulates the body to rest and digest – heart rate decreases, breathing slows, digestion increases and the body's energy supplies are maintained.[12] Just as we react to negative stimuli that are harmful, we also instinctively react to positive stimuli – such as water and vegetation – that aid survival or promote wellbeing. Ulrich proposes that everyday natural settings can provide a valuable "breather" from stress as they can promote more positive emotions and revitalize energy levels.[12, 25, 27] Indeed, studies have found that viewing nature enhances activity of the parasympathetic nervous system, helping with recovery from stress.[56]

ATTENTION RESTORATION THEORY (ART)

ART was proposed by Rachel and Stephen Kaplan[57] in 1989 and is based on the restoration of "directed attention". Trying to maintain intense concentration (directed attention) for any period of time can be mentally exhausting. As we increasingly struggle to concentrate, we may become impatient, irritable and easily distracted and, before long, we need to take a break.[58] It is suggested that our mental fatigue could be reduced by spending time in, or even simply viewing, a "restorative environment". We find nature intrinsically fascinating and therefore viewing interesting natural environments takes no effort. This effortless attention allows our brains to rest and mentally recover. For an environment to be "restorative", they propose that it contains four key components:[59]

1. **Fascination** – some aspects of the environment must hold one's attention effortlessly. "Soft" fascination is thought to be the most important component: softly fascinating stimuli, such as waves breaking on the shore, require little attention and enable mental reflection.

2. **Being Away** – there must be an element of "getting away from it all". The environment must be psychologically or physically removed from a person's daily routine.

3. **Extent** – the environment must have enough content and structure that it feels like being "immersed" in another world.

4. **Compatibility** – it should be an environment that a person wishes to be exposed to and engage with.

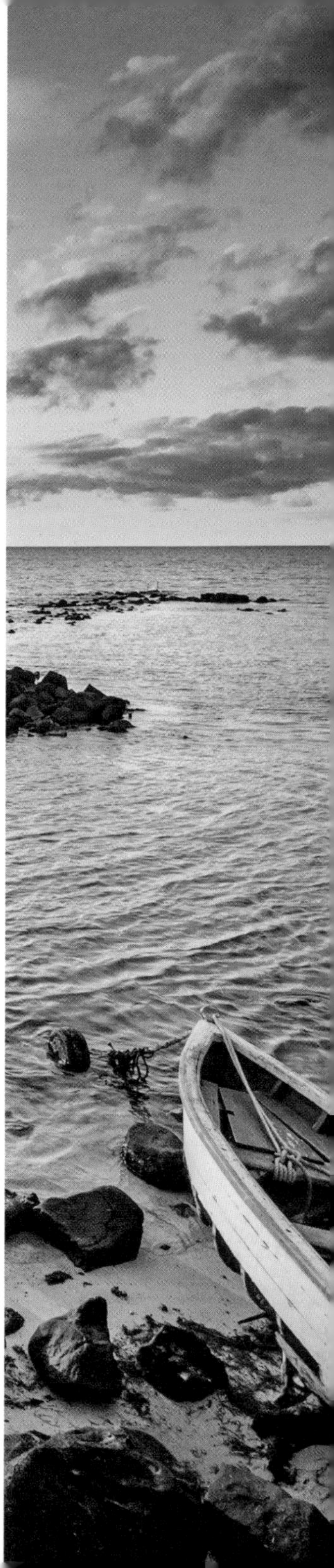

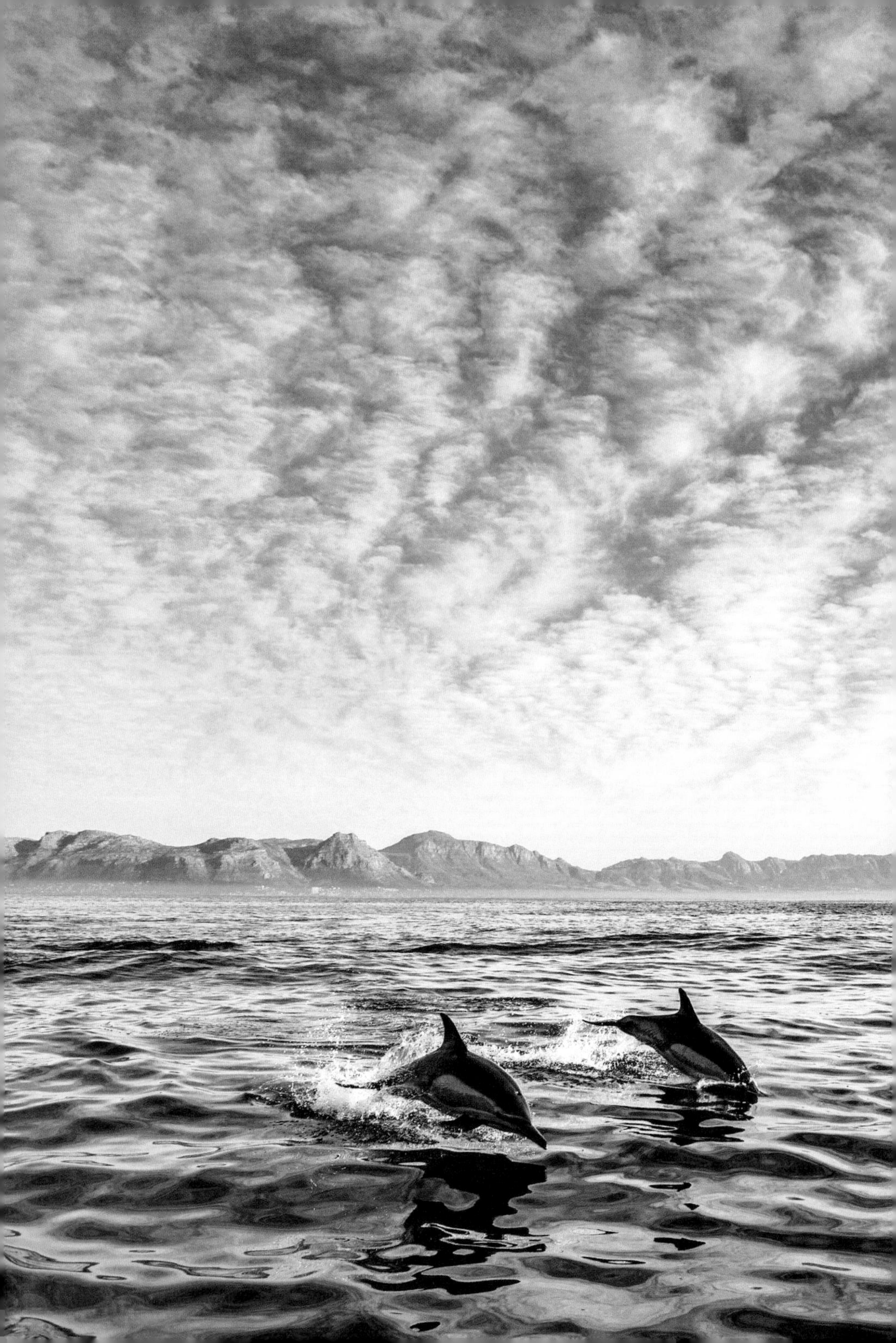

An Introduction to Environmental Psychology

The study of how restorative environments influence human health and wellbeing is just one topic of research in the interdisciplinary field known as "environmental psychology". Although the exact origins of this field are unknown, Willy Hugo Hellpach is often credited with being the first to use the term "environmental psychology" in the early 20th century[60]. Broadly speaking, environmental psychologists are interested in the positive and negative interactions between individuals and their surroundings.[61] We are always somewhere – at home, in school, at work, in public spaces, or natural environments – and environmental psychology research covers all of these social, informational, learning, built, and natural settings.

The range of research undertaken by environmental psychologists is vast. For instance, they may study our online shopping habits, how we are affected by crowding and noise, how we use social media, what makes us feel safer on the streets or more productive in the office, what influences our pro-environmental behaviours or how we interact in virtual environments.

As all aspects of human existence occur in one setting or another, it is critical that we fully understand the relationships between people and their environment. While our surroundings shape us – affecting how we feel and act – we also shape the land, air, water and other forms of life around us. Therefore, a greater understanding of these complex interactions is important for people, and their natural and built surroundings.[61]

The Relationship Between Mankind and the Oceans

As discussed on pages 31–3, we can be greatly affected – both positively and negatively – by our surroundings. The pressures of modern living, especially in busy, urban environments, can introduce stress into our lives on a daily basis. Being exposed to nature can provide an antidote, positively influencing our health and wellbeing. While many theories and studies have focused on green space – arguably, the most accessible form of nature – I wish to highlight the benefits of a less well-researched topic: the benefits of blue space and, specifically, the sea.

The following four chapters will discuss the benefits we can derive from the oceans, both physical and mental, including how we can optimize these benefits while we are by the sea, and how we can enjoy those benefits closer to home. However, in the final chapter, on pages 152–81, I wish to shift the focus away from how we can benefit from the oceans, to how the oceans can benefit from us.

We live in deeply troubling times. Almost every day, we hear about the harmful impacts human actions are having on the oceans. While the oceans provide us with many health and wellbeing benefits, they are not there for our sole and unconditional use. We are part of nature and all of nature is interlinked in a complex and co-dependent web: we can never be fully sure how our actions today will ultimately affect the balance of such delicate natural systems. It is our responsibility to maintain the health of the oceans for the sake of everyone and everything on our planet.

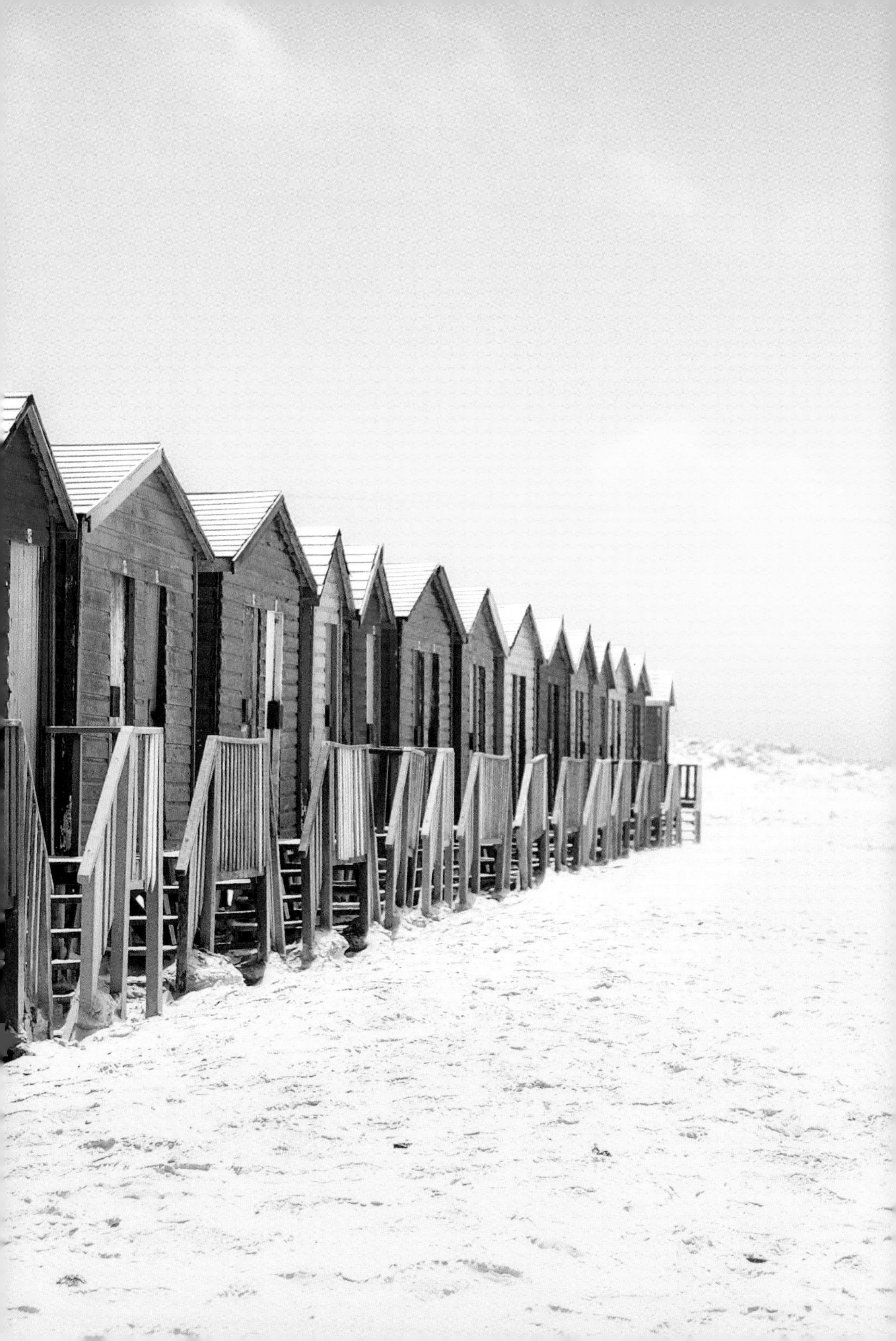

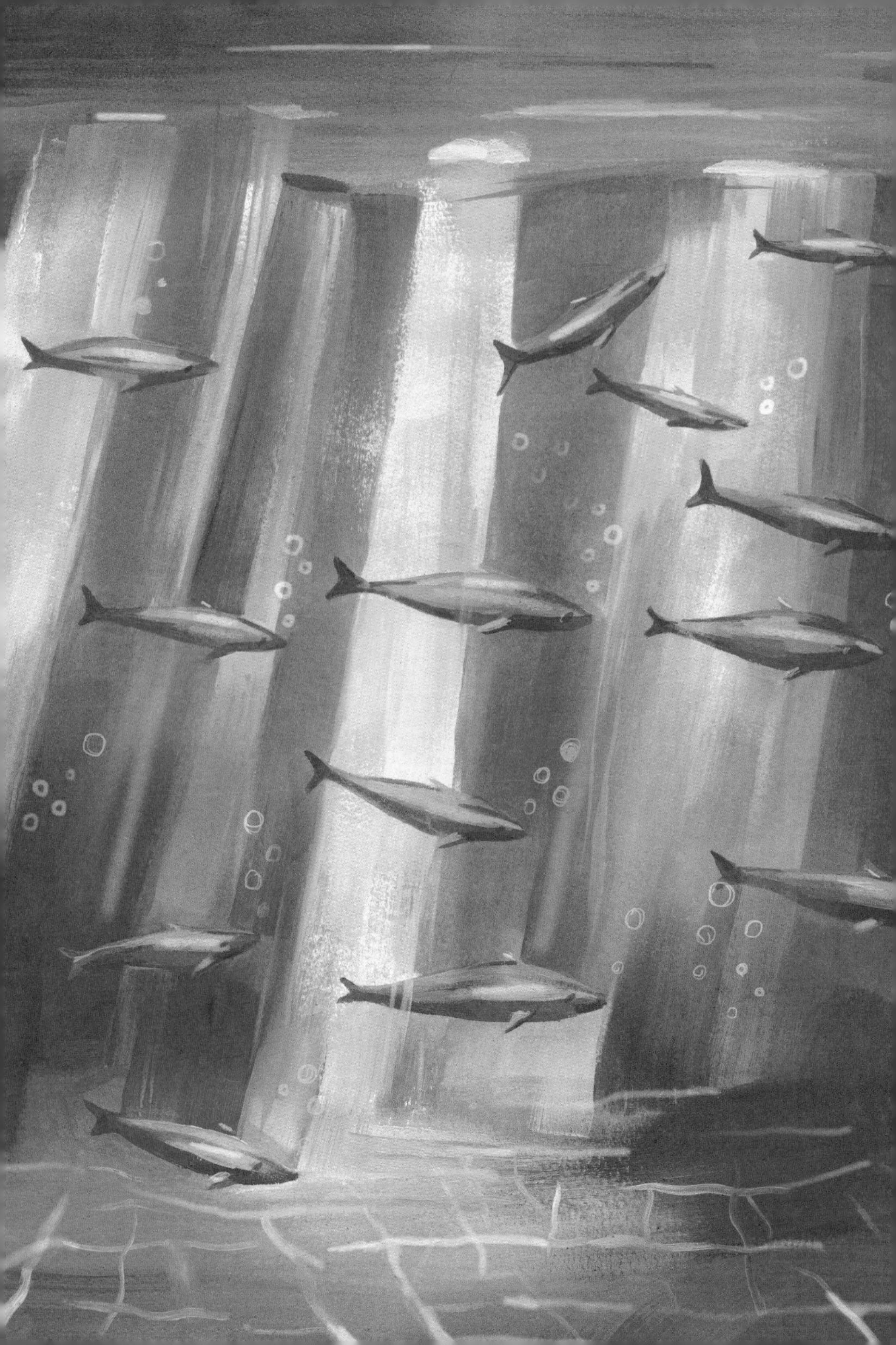

CHAPTER 2

The Physical Benefits of the Sea

"My soul is full of longing
For the secret of the sea,
And the heart of the great ocean
Sends a thrilling pulse through me."

— Henry Wadsworth Longfellow

The marine environment provides us with many positive benefits for health and wellbeing. It is a source of nutritious food; a provider of important pharmaceuticals; a location that promotes physical activity and valuable opportunities to spend time with family and friends; and a setting that can help calm our thoughts and restore our busy minds. While keeping in mind that physical and mental health are inextricably linked, this chapter outlines some of the many physical health benefits the sea can offer us.

SEAFOOD

Fish and shellfish are good sources of protein, the building blocks for our bodies' muscles, bones and organs (see pages 144–5). Seafood also provides valuable vitamins – such as vitamins A and D – and minerals, including iodine which is important for thyroid function. Oily fish, such as mackerel and tuna, are especially high in omega-3 fatty acids which have been found to be beneficial in preventing or mitigating a range of common diseases and conditions, including coronary heart disease and stroke,[62] osteoarthritis, rheumatoid arthritis, inflammatory bowel diseases (such as Crohn's disease), age-related macular degeneration and skin conditions like eczema.

Seaweeds (marine macroalgae) are another source of important omega-3 fatty acids (see pages 150–1). Seaweed is also low in calories and saturated fat, yet rich in vitamins, minerals, protein and fibre. It can provide us with many nutritional health benefits, especially when compared with many terrestrial plant and animal-based foods.[63, 64]

PHARMACEUTICALS

As well as providing nutritional benefits, compounds derived from seaweeds and other marine organisms (such as molluscs, corals and sponges) provide valuable new medicines and pharmaceuticals. Over 6,000 unique compounds have been isolated from marine organisms, with hundreds showing therapeutic properties. Marine sponges, in particular, are considered one of the richest sources of potential new

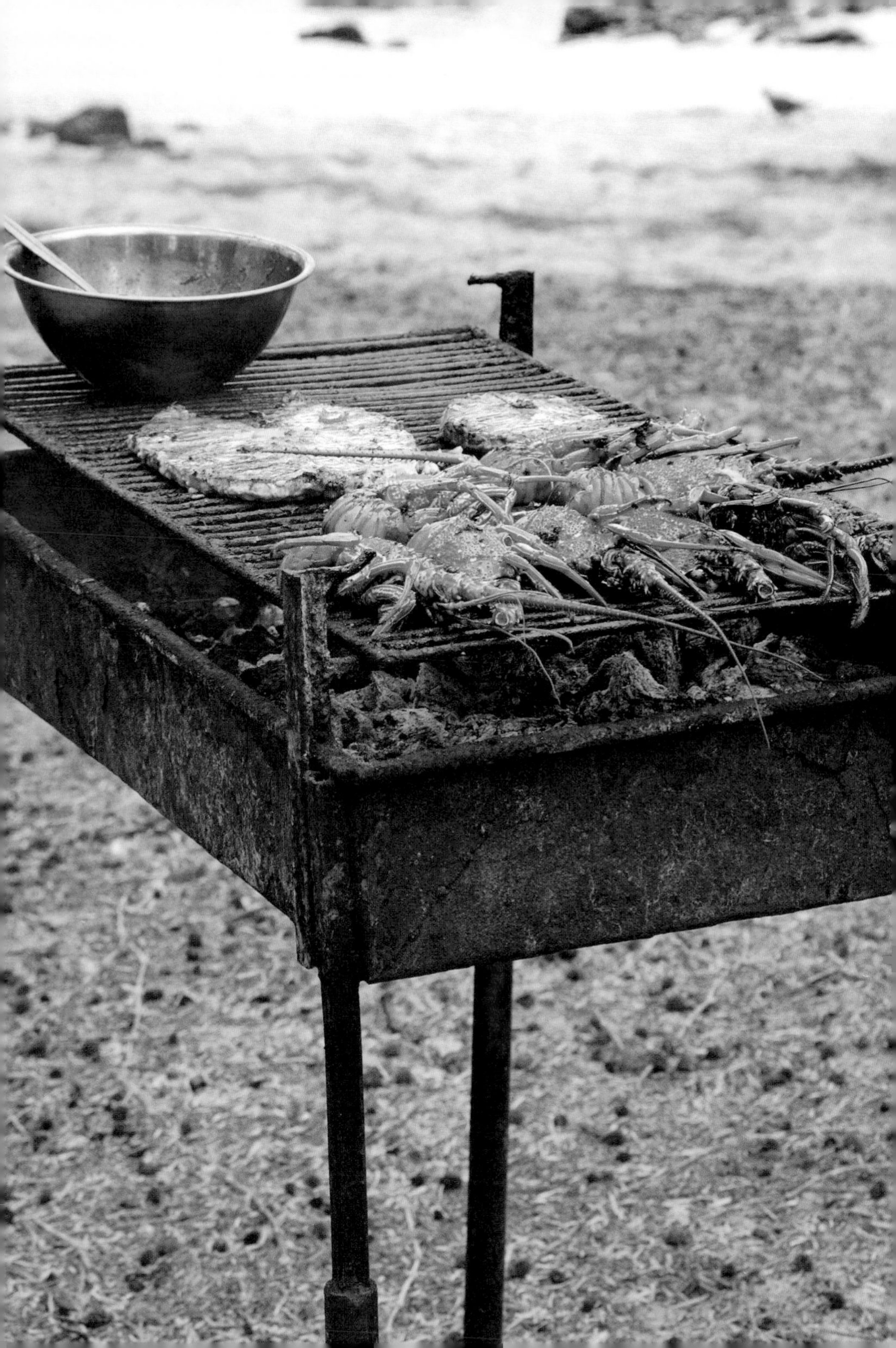

pharmaceuticals. Studies on compounds derived from marine sponges have revealed many important therapeutic properties, including antibacterial, antiviral, antifungal, anticancer, anti-inflammatory and antimalarial.[63, 65–67]

The Problems of Antimicrobial Resistance

Antimicrobial medicines are used to prevent and treat infections caused by microorganisms, such as bacteria, viruses and fungi. When microorganisms change their response to these drugs (such as antibiotics), antimicrobial resistance occurs and the infection can no longer be treated. More and more microorganisms are becoming drug resistant and a growing number of infections, such as tuberculosis and pneumonia, are becoming more difficult to treat.

Antimicrobial resistance not only threatens human health (around 700,000 people die of antimicrobial-resistant infections each year) but impacts animals and crops, affecting food security and safety. There is, therefore, an urgent need to discover new antimicrobials, and compounds derived from marine sponges may help.[68, 69]

Thalassotherapy and Related Treatments

Although scientists continue to search for valuable new compounds to help combat some of the most serious diseases and illnesses of our time, marine organisms, along with sea water and fresh sea air, have been used throughout history to treat problems with our physical health.

Thalassotherapy (from *thalassa*, the Greek word for "sea") uses seawater, products from the sea (such as seaweeds), and the marine environment itself, as a form of therapy. Some of the earliest accounts of thalassotherapy originate from ancient civilizations, including the Greeks, Romans and Egyptians, who used seawater for a range of ailments.[66]

However, around the mid-1700s, it was Doctor Richard Russell, a British physician, who highlighted the potential benefits of thalassotherapy. After reviewing numerous case studies, Russell concluded that the minerals found in seawater (such as magnesium and other trace elements) could help treat a variety of medical conditions.[7] Russell started a practice in Brighton and sea bathing became extremely popular. Hospitals were established by the sea in other parts of England and interest spread to Europe, where thalassotherapy centres flourished during the 19th century, particularly in France and Germany. Robust scientific evidence of the benefits was however lacking, and the introduction of antibiotics in the mid-20th century saw a decline in the use of thalassotherapy as a medical treatment.[70]

More recently in Western societies, "traditional" medical approaches (such as acupuncture, herbalism and homeopathy) are becoming increasingly popular as an alternative to conventional medicine. There may be several reasons for this interest in alternative and complementary medicines, including a dissatisfaction with conventional healthcare due to the adverse effects of some modern medicines, their inefficiency for certain conditions and long waiting lists. There is also a perception that "natural" alternatives may be more effective and safer.[71] This renewed interest in such alternative medicines has prompted the re-emergence of thalassotherapy.[7]

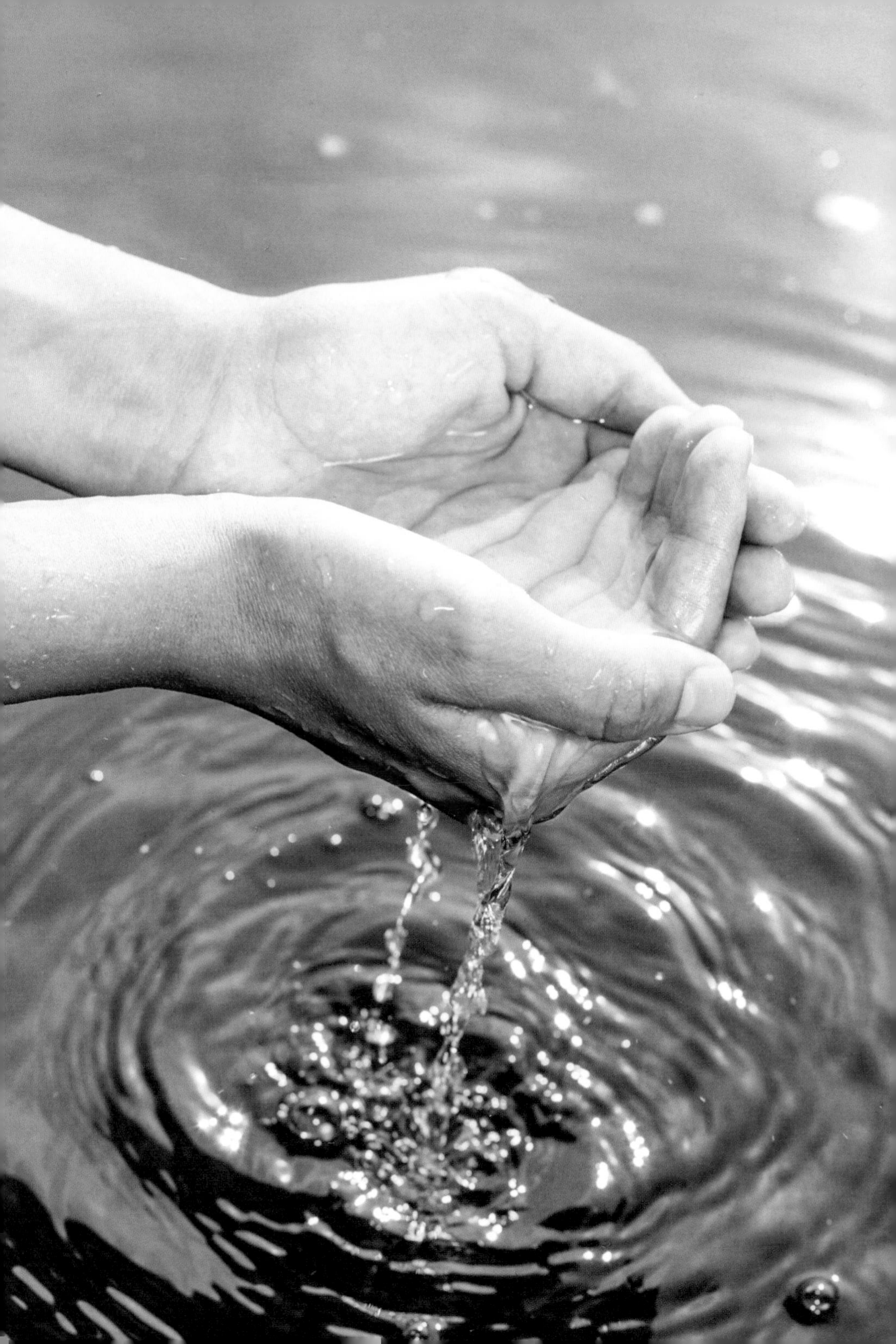

DOES THALASSOTHERAPY WORK?

Although there appears some disagreement on the effectiveness of magnesium absorption through the skin, compared with oral supplementation,[72,73] sea bathing has long been regarded as an additional source of magnesium. It is believed that salt water is good for treating a variety of conditions, particularly skin conditions such as eczema.

Beauty spas offer many sea-based treatments that have their roots in thalassotherapy, such as seaweed wraps that are thought to draw toxins and excess fluid from the body, helping conditions like cellulite build-up. While it is likely that researchers will continue to investigate these various treatments and products to determine their effectiveness, there already appears increasing evidence that thalassotherapy and related treatments may be beneficial for several ailments, including arthritis, rheumatism and back pain.[66]

Some also argue that perhaps a lack of scientifically robust evidence of the effectiveness of alternative treatments (such as spa treatments or aromatherapy) should not necessarily preclude them from use. There is often very little rigorous, hard evidence in support of complementary and alternative therapies, yet those who use them still report benefiting from these treatments. It is suggested, therefore, that if a therapy has no adverse effects and helps people through its powerful "placebo" effect then perhaps is should be used irrespective of clinical evidence.[7,71]

THE BENEFITS OF TAKING THE SEA AIR

Respiratory problems are also thought to benefit from the coastal environment. Indeed, breathing fresh, clean air has long been associated with good health – even today health service websites suggest that a good supply of fresh air is beneficial for helping to prevent the spread of tuberculosis.[74] Research suggests that sea air may be especially beneficial. Alongside anecdotal evidence suggesting that ocean air helped to clear the lungs of surfers suffering with cystic fibrosis, researchers found that inhaling an intensely salty solution helped to improve lung function and lessen other complications of the disease.[75]

Physical Activity

The most vigorous aspect of sea bathing – physical exercise – could be considered one of the main benefits of being by the sea. Lack of physical activity can increase the risk of many physical health problems – including cardiovascular disease, high blood pressure, obesity and diabetes – as well as being detrimental to our mental health. So adequate physical activity is important for maintaining both our physical and mental health over our lifetime.[22]

Research suggests that natural environments may influence how physically active we are by providing opportunities for certain types of activities. Furthermore, exercising in natural settings may provide health benefits above and beyond physical activity alone.[22] In terms of general wellbeing, exercising in a natural environment improves self-esteem, boosts confidence and improves mood, in particular reducing tension, anger and depression. People are also more likely to want to repeat the exercise than those who have worked out indoors. Interestingly, the first five minutes of such exercise appears to have the biggest impact on mood and self-esteem, suggesting an immediate psychological health benefit.[76]

On a physical level, your workout or walk might just feel that little bit easier if you are doing it outside. One study found that when they were allowed to choose their own walking speed, participants tended to walk faster outdoors compared to indoors. And paradoxically, they reported that they felt they had put in less effort.[77]

When asked to put in the same amount of exertion to a walk indoors and outdoors, individuals tended to walk faster outdoors, using greater physiological effort, which suggests they found the exercise to be less demanding when performed in a natural environment.[78] The theory is that being surrounded by a pleasant environment reduces our awareness of physiological sensations and negative emotions, thus minimizing the feeling of effort. This allows us to put in more effort and for longer, which may help to increase the amount of exercise we do and the motivation to continue.

BLUE EXERCISE AND THE "BLUE GYM"

Many early studies explored how green spaces could help promote physical activity and in the mid-1990s the "Green Gym" initiative was established. The aim was to enable people who would not usually attend a sports centre or gym to improve their fitness and wellbeing while also taking care of their green spaces through conservation activities.[79]

More recently, we have seen the establishment of the "Blue Gym" initiative. Based on the Green Gym idea, the Blue Gym initiative has two main aims:

- To understand the potential for "natural" aquatic settings (such as lakes, rivers and coastlines) to promote and enhance human health and wellbeing.
- To increase public awareness of marine issues, encouraging people to protect and preserve these fragile environments.

This has lead to many new research studies investigating the health benefits of "blue exercise", and has also inspired people to engage with natural blue spaces in a more responsible way.[47]

Blue exercise is a physical activity undertaken in or around any natural blue space.[80] These activities may be in the water (for example swimming), on the water (for example surfing, kayaking or paddleboarding), under the water (for example scuba diving), or simply by the water (for example walking along the beach). While the term "blue exercise" may be relatively new, we can presume that humans have been exercising in and around water for hundreds, if not thousands, of years.

Throughout history, water has been used, primarily, as a source of food or as a means of transport, yet some activities, such as riding the ocean waves, developed into a pastime and were doubtless also undertaken for pleasure. Although accurate ancient records of wave riding may be difficult to establish, the first Westerners to observe surfing were Captain James Cook and the crew on the

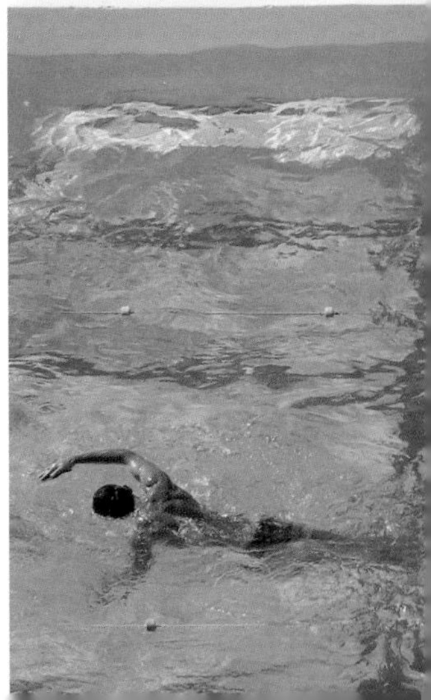

HMS *Endeavour*, during their stay on the Polynesian island of Tahiti in the late 1770s.[81]

Around this time, medicinal sea bathing (thalassotherapy) became popular and was often followed by a brisk stroll along the beach to maximize intake of the invigorating sea air. By the mid-1800s the focus broadened from sea bathing for purely medicinal purposes to include recreational swimming for exercise and enjoyment.[47] Increased leisure time and improved access to the coast during the 1900s fuelled interest in using the coast and ocean for recreation and pleasure. Today, in the 21st century, although many people cite relaxation and social motivations for being by the sea, the physical activities undertaken at the beach and along the coast are not without merit.[82]

THE BENEFITS OF BLUE EXERCISE

Physical activity can help reduce a person's risk of developing many major illnesses, such as heart disease, stroke and type-2 diabetes. The risk of some cancers can be reduced by up to 50 per cent and the risk of early death can be lowered by up to 30 per cent. Exercise can boost self-esteem, lift mood, increase energy levels and improve sleep quality. It can also help reduce the risk of stress and depression, as well as dementia and Alzheimer's disease.[74]

According to the UK's National Health Service (NHS) website, it has been medically proven that people who do regular physical activity have:

- up to a 35 per cent lower risk of coronary heart disease and stroke
- up to a 50 per cent lower risk of type-2 diabetes
- up to a 50 per cent lower risk of colon cancer
- up to a 20 per cent lower risk of breast cancer

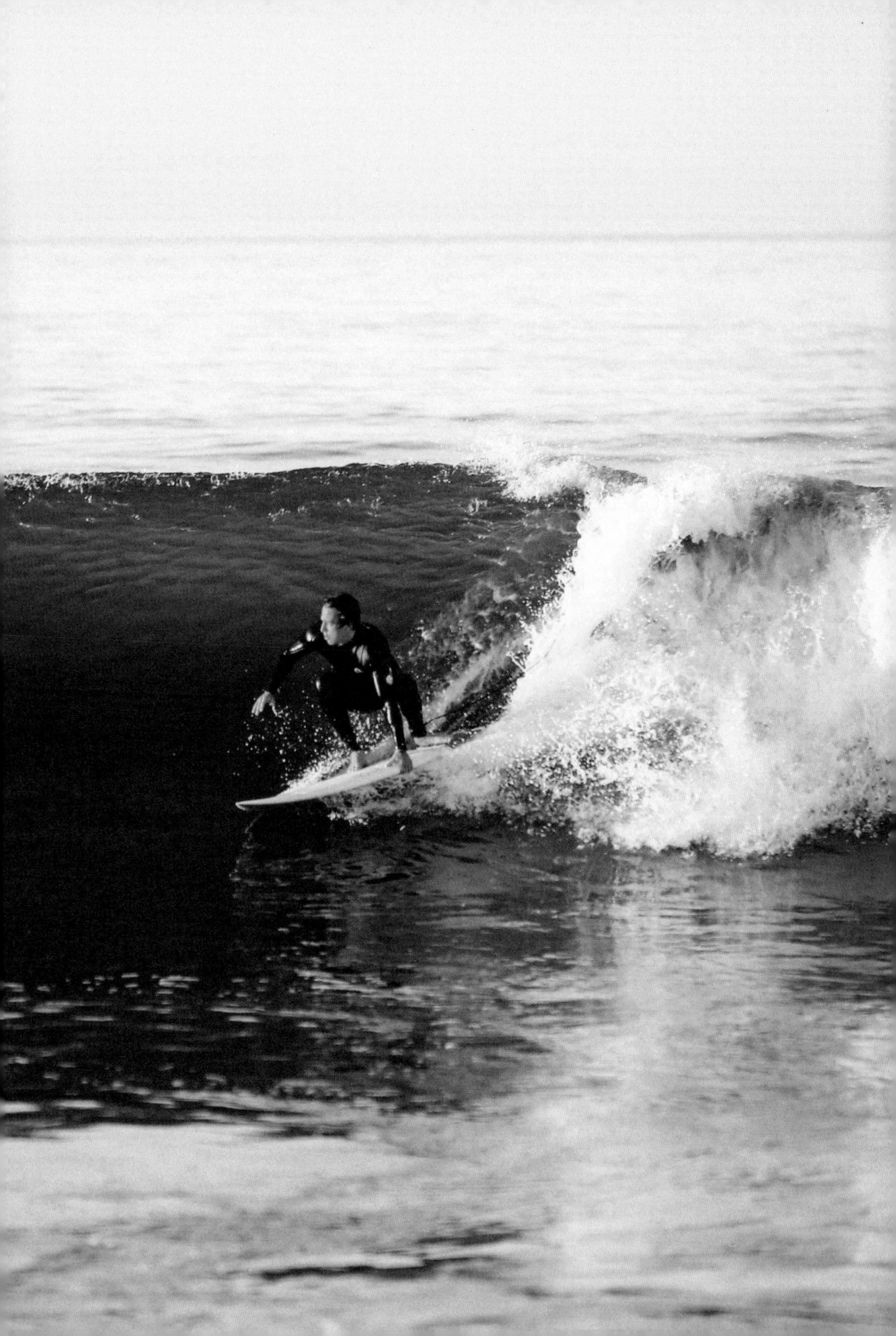

- a 30 per cent lower risk of early death
- up to an 83 per cent lower risk of osteoarthritis
- up to a 68 per cent lower risk of hip fracture
- a 30 per cent lower risk of falls among older adults
- up to a 30 per cent lower risk of depression
- up to a 30 per cent lower risk of dementia

Research has found that people who live closer to the sea tend to be happier and healthier than people who live further inland.[3] It is thought that one reason for this may be because living nearer to the coast encourages higher levels of physical activity, resulting in the multiple health benefits described.[83] Studies in New Zealand and Australia found a relationship between living near the sea and self-reported rates of physical activity. A UK-based study also broadly supported the Australasian findings, revealing that a person was more likely to meet the recommended level of physical activity if they lived closer to the coast.[83]

TYPES OF BLUE EXERCISE

So what sorts of activities do we undertake when at the coast? Research suggests that by far the most popular activity is walking. Walking is a great activity because it is free, involves no specialist equipment, can be taken at any pace, and has relatively low impact on the joints. Brisk walking at 3–4mph (5–6.5kph) is classed as moderately intense physical activity and is especially beneficial.[84]

Although not as popular as walking, activities of higher or lower intensity still provide benefits. Higher-intensity activities – such as swimming, canoeing and surfing – provide greater cardiovascular benefits than lower-intensity activities such as angling,[85] but lower-intensity activities provide benefits if undertaken often enough. For instance, angling is classed as a low to moderate physical activity, yet some people like to go angling many times throughout the year, compared with a higher-intensity activity such as coasteering which they may do only infrequently.[86] Furthermore, as visits to the coast tend to last longer than visits to other environments, even less intense activities could result in a considerable amount of physical activity in the long term.[85]

LAND VS SEA ACTIVITIES

Exercising in water is becoming increasingly popular. Water provides buoyancy and creates resistance, resulting in aerobic exercise with relatively little impact or strain on the joints, yet requiring high levels of energy. Water-based exercise may be especially suitable for certain groups of people, such as the elderly and those with orthopaedic problems, back pain, arthritis, osteoporosis, or any other medical conditions that training on land may limit. Furthermore, water resistance increases the energy cost of certain exercises: walking in waist-high water will be more strenuous that walking at the same speed on a treadmill.[87]

POOL VS SEA EXERCISE

One study compared how women with fibromyalgia (a long-term condition that causes pain throughout the body) responded to the same aerobic exercise programme performed either in a water pool or the sea. The researchers found that, although exercising in water was effective for both groups, those that exercised in the sea enjoyed greater emotional benefits.[88]

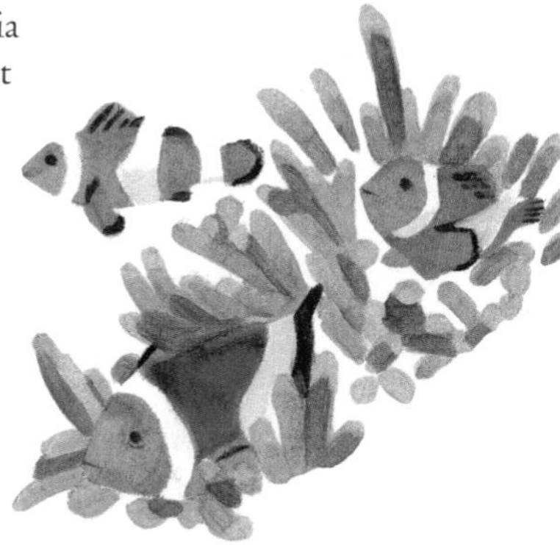

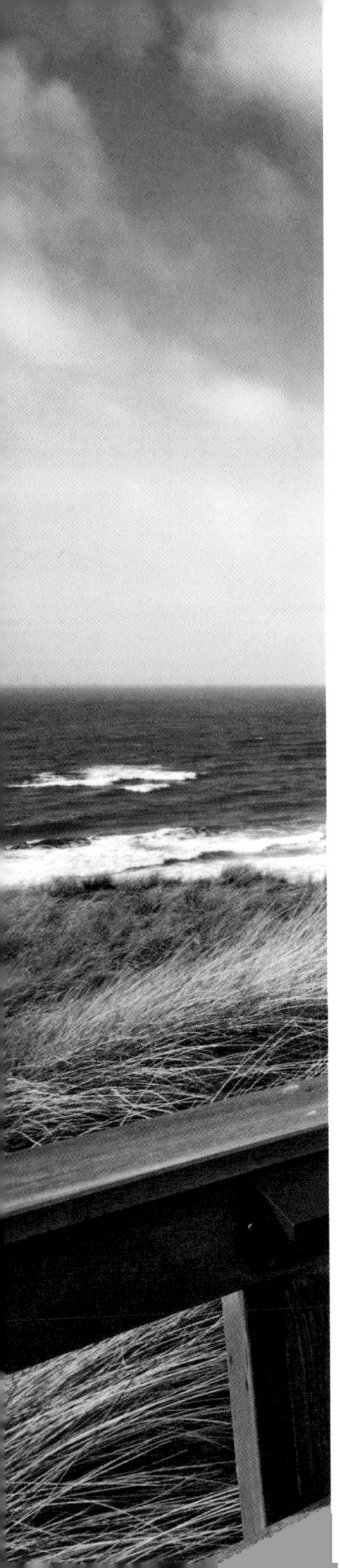

HOW BLUE SPACE CAN BOOST FAMILY EXERCISE

It is thought that families, especially, may benefit from time at the seaside. Using in-depth interviews with families with children aged 8–11, researchers in the UK found that children saw the beach as a place where the whole family were more likely to play together. For instance, in other outdoor spaces such as parks, adults tended to sit on a bench watching the children play but at the beach, adults were more likely to get up and play football, frisbee or go swimming as a family. In addition to increased physical exercise, other health benefits included experiencing fun, feeling less stressed, and enjoying the social interaction that family time at the beach brought.[6]

HOW BLUE EXERCISE CAN HELP COMBAT LIFE CHALLENGES

Learning outside the classroom (LOTC) – allowing children to learn through experiences beyond the classroom[89] – is thought to be an important way to complement classroom-based learning. Outdoor activities can be an important LOTC tool, especially for children and young people who are at risk of exclusion, or have already been excluded, from mainstream schooling. One study evaluated the impact of a bespoke 12-week surfing programme on one such group of 12–16 year olds. The programme taught the young people how to surf and provided information on environmental issues and sustainability.

Researchers found that after the programme, there was a significant drop in heart rate compared with pre-programme levels, suggesting an improvement in fitness. Engaging in blue exercise programmes also resulted in other benefits, such as more positive attitudes toward school and friendships, and greater environmental awareness.[90] Although not always rigorously researched, evaluation of similar programmes (such as sailing weeks), indicates that vulnerable children gain physical, mental and social benefits from engaging in blue space activities.

Anecdotal evidence suggests that adults, too, can benefit from such programmes. Offering sailing, kayaking and surfing activities, organizations in the UK and abroad can help people with physical disabilities (such as amputations) and psychological issues (such as post-traumatic stress disorder (PTSD), depression or addiction), overcome their particular life challenges. It is suggested that those suffering from drug and alcohol addiction may particularly benefit from activities such as surfing, competitive paddleboard racing and whitewater kayaking. It is thought that these activities provide an alternative "high", thus "satisfying the brain's desire for stimulation, novelty, and neurochemical 'rush'".[91]

CAN BEING BY THE SEA PROMOTE PHYSICAL ACTIVITY?

Many people find it difficult to gain the benefits of physical activity: some common reasons given are a lack of time, insufficient motivation and a dislike of exercise because it's uncomfortable, boring or futile. There are, however, other factors that determine a person's likelihood and motivation to exercise, such as gender, age and socio-economic classification. For instance, research suggests that young girls tend to be less physically active than boys,[92] and that females are more likely to exercise for weight loss and body toning than males, who tend to exercise more for enjoyment.[93]

So, can being by the sea influence some of these factors? Using data collected over seven years as part of the Monitor of Engagement with the Natural Environment (MENE) survey, researchers looked at how 326,755 English residents spent their leisure time in different natural settings, such as beaches, the coast, inland water bodies (such as rivers, lakes, canals), urban parks, and wooded

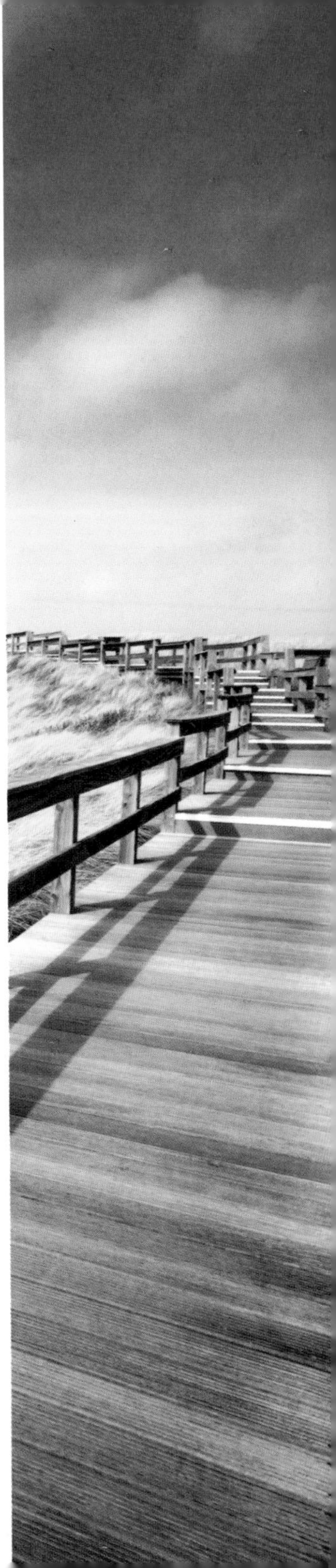

and forested areas.[85] Researchers found that although people tended to visit beaches and the coast less often than other settings (presumably because other environments, such as urban parks, are easier to access), visits to these settings were of extreme importance, especially for certain members of society. For instance, visits to coastal environments were more likely to be undertaken by females, and older adults. As these two groups of people are normally less physically active than males or younger adults, they suggest that visits to the coast could be a good way to encourage these less active groups to get more exercise.

Interestingly, when asked why they visited natural environments, people visiting coastal settings mentioned that they did so for social reasons (such as spending time with the family) or to relax and unwind. Going to the coast for health and exercise was mentioned less often.[85] However, considering that physical activity, especially walking, still usually takes place during these coastal visits, this could actually be a good thing. Some people may struggle with the concept of "exercise", thinking it means spending hours each day in a gym, running and lifting weights, but if being by the sea can indirectly encourage physical activity through walking with friends or playing on the beach, then people will be exercising without necessarily realizing it.

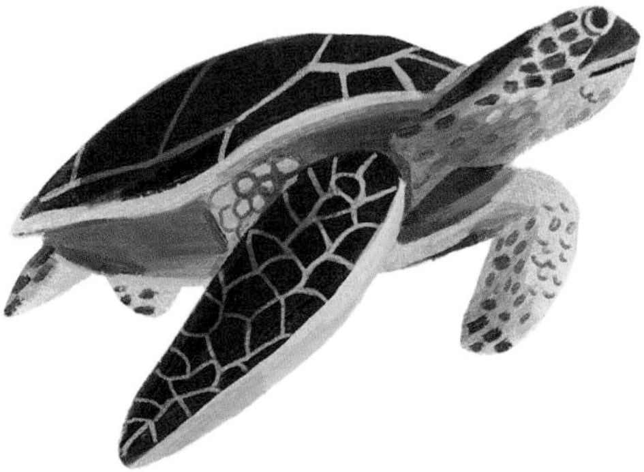

Blue Zones

Blue Zones are places in the world where people live a particularly long time. The phrase "Blue Zones" is associated with journalist and author Dan Buettner, whose cover story, "The Secrets of a Long Life", was publish in *National Geographic* magazine in 2005. Research in Sardinia had previously established the highest concentration of male centenarians[94] and Buettner identified five regions where people statistically live much longer than average:

- Okinawa (Japan)
- Sardinia (Italy)
- Nicoya Peninsula (Costa Rica)
- Icaria (Greece)
- Loma Linda, a community of Adventists (USA)

Buettner also established that, not only did these regions have high numbers of people over 100 years old, but that many had grown old without the health problems that commonly affect people in the developed world, such as obesity, diabetes, heart disease and cancer. People that live in Blue Zones share many lifestyle characteristics, including staying moderately physically active, putting family ahead of other concerns, and having a social circle. Being by the sea can help foster many of these characteristics. The beach cities of Southern California have secured funding for a Blue Zone Project, which not only focuses on physical health but on community interaction, including walking, fitness and mindfulness activities.[95]

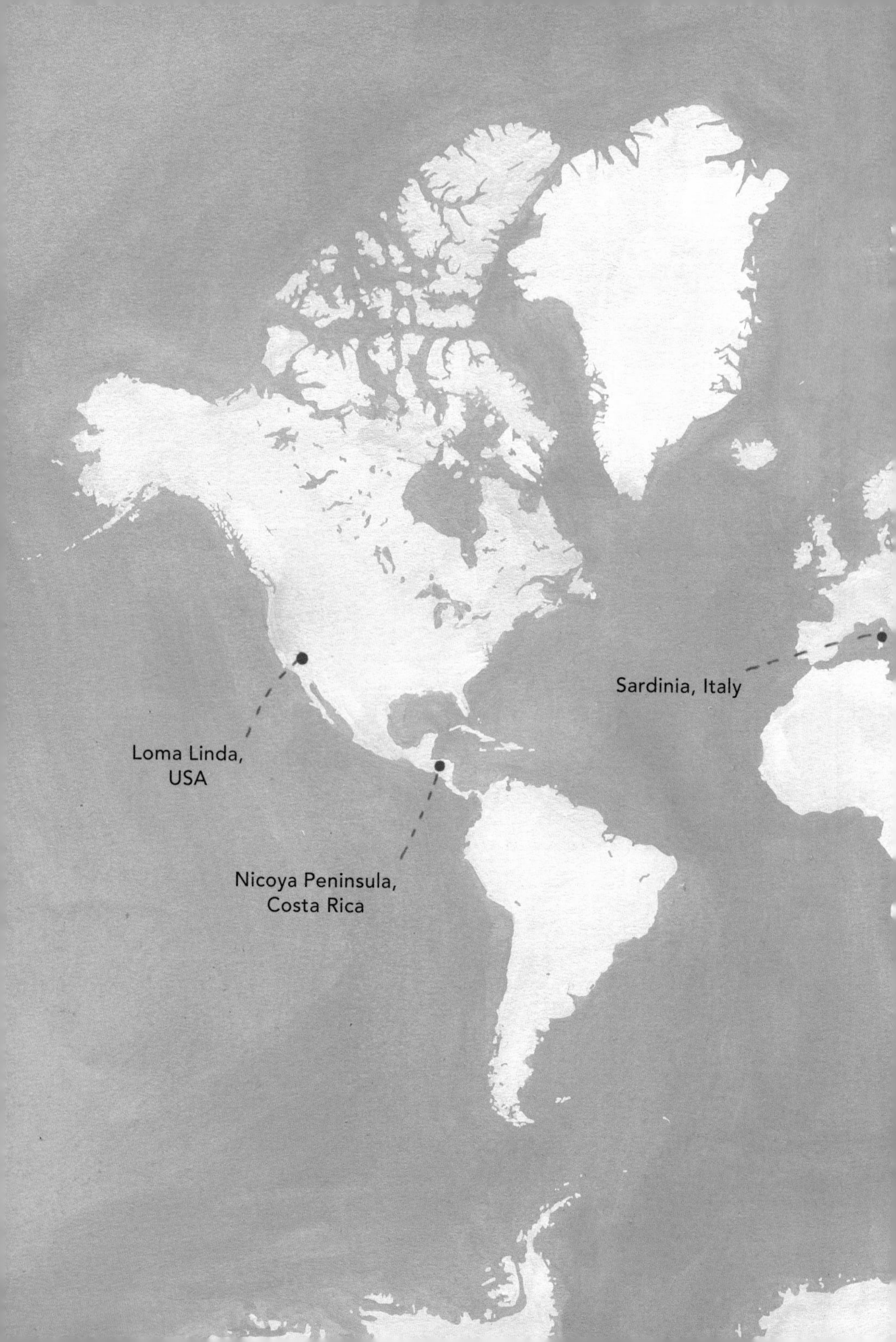
Sardinia, Italy
Loma Linda,
USA
Nicoya Peninsula,
Costa Rica

The Blue Zones

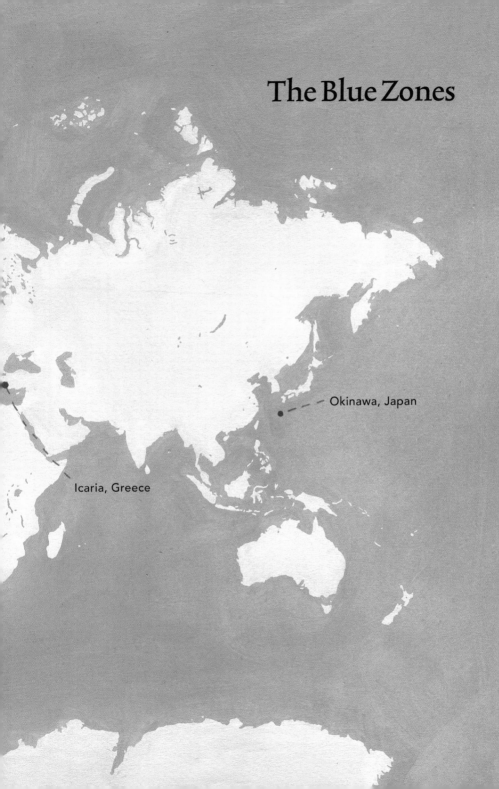

Better Sleep

As well as being a beneficial physical activity, walking at the coast provides an opportunity to breathe in the fresh sea air, which many people believe promotes a better night's sleep. Sufficient, good-quality sleep is essential for health and wellbeing, and insufficient or poor-quality sleep is associated with:

- an increased risk of weight gain and obesity in children and adults
- poor concentration, productivity and performance
- poor athletic and physical performance
- an increased risk of chronic diseases, including heart disease and stroke
- adverse effects on blood sugar levels, increasing the risk of type-2 diabetes
- mental health issues, especially depression
- impaired immune function
- inflammatory problems within the body, such as inflammatory bowel disease
- adverse effects on emotions and social interaction.[96]

Seeking to learn a little more about the link between a coastal walk and improved sleep, one study compared how walkers in two different types of natural environment (the coast versus inland), felt after their walks. Just over a hundred walkers, between the ages of 21 and 82, walked for approximately 7 miles (11km), either along a coast path or inland through hills, heathland and parks. Both groups of walkers reported that they felt calmer, happier and more alert after their walks. They also slept better and for longer. However, the coast path walkers slept significantly longer than walkers taking the inland routes, sleeping on average an extra 47 minutes per night.

Why might this be? In this study, walking by the coast was more likely to bring back previous memories (such as childhood holidays by the sea), than inland walks. Thinking back to the theories surrounding restorative environments, potentially these enhanced feelings of being away from daily routines may have contributed to a greater restorative experience than walking inland,[97] resulting in better and longer sleep. It is more likely that a combination of the restorative effect of viewing the sea, breathing fresh air, together with a reasonable amount of exercise, helps promote a better night's sleep.

What Are Negative Ions and Do They Benefit Health?

Negative ions are generated in nature as air molecules are broken apart by sunlight or the movement of air and water. They are, therefore, abundant in natural locations such as beaches and waterfalls. Many people believe that negative ions may be beneficial for health by improving mood, relieving stress and aiding sleep. Overall, there appears little, if any, scientific evidence to support claims that negative ions in natural environments are beneficial for physical health but negative-ion-generating devices can significantly improve indoor air quality, by removing fine particles, airborne microbials and some harmful volatile organic compounds, as well as neutralizing odours.[98] Furthermore, there is some evidence to suggest that negative ionization, particularly at high-density levels, has a positive effect on depression.[99]

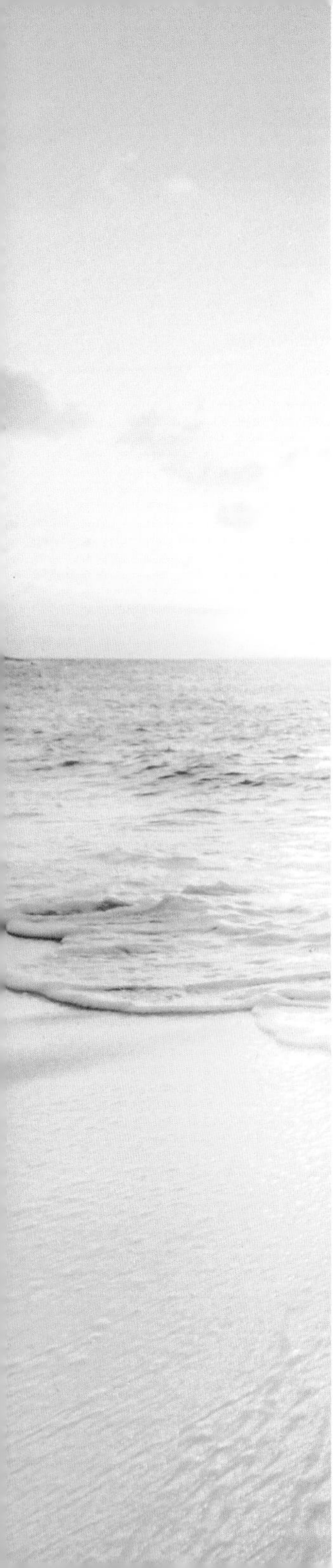

Vitamin D – the Sunshine Vitamin

Another benefit of being by the sea is our exposure to direct sunlight, the main source of ultraviolet radiation, which naturally produces vitamin D in our skin. Vitamin D, the "sunshine vitamin", has several important functions. Although usually associated with bone health – one of its most critical functions is to regulate the amount of calcium and phosphate in the body, vital for healthy bones, teeth and muscle[100] – vitamin D is also known for its importance to our immune system, our digestive health and our mental wellbeing, not to mention its anticancer properties.[101–103]

VITAMIN D AND IMMUNITY

Our immune system defends our bodies from attack by foreign organisms and promotes protective immunity. It also maintains our tolerance to our own bodies – our immune system can normally tell the difference between our own cells and foreign cells. However, if our body's immune system fails to recognize its own tissues and cells, it can attack the body as if it were a foreign or invading organism. This autoimmunity can cause a variety of human illnesses, such as type-1 diabetes, psoriasis, rheumatoid arthritis and lupus. Vitamin D deficiency is associated with increased autoimmunity and susceptibility to infection.[104]

Insufficient vitamin D levels have also been associated with an increase in risk of metabolic syndrome (MetS), a set of conditions that includes abdominal obesity, high blood pressure, abnormal cholesterol, and high blood sugar levels (which, left unchecked, can lead to type-2 diabetes). Having any of these conditions can affect the blood vessels, but having all three together increases the risk of serious health problems, such as heart disease and stroke.[105] A Brazilian study found MetS in almost two-thirds of post-menopausal women with a vitamin D deficiency, but in less than 40 per cent of those who had sufficient vitamin D levels.[106]

VITAMIN D, CANCER AND DIGESTIVE HEALTH

Research has already established a link between insufficient vitamin D levels and an increased risk of certain cancers, such as prostate, breast and ovarian.[107] We know that vitamin D has powerful anticancer properties, particularly against digestive-system cancers.[108]

Vitamin D deficiency is also linked to poor digestive health: many people suffering from debilitating disorders of the gastrointestinal tract, such as inflammatory bowel disease (IBD) and irritable bowel syndrome (IBS), are vitamin D deficient. IBS affects 20 per cent of the UK population and accounts for 10 per cent of visits to GP surgeries. It is thought that getting sufficient vitamin D (for example through supplementation) may help ease symptoms.[103]

As vitamin D is only found in a small number of foods, access to direct sunlight is an important source (although obviously care should be taken not to overexpose, as too much unprotected sun exposure can increase the risk of skin cancers). Studies have found that ultraviolet radiation tends to be greater at the coast because of the effects that the landscape has on the clouds – put simply, more sunshine gets through. In northern Europe, this is especially important in the autumn and winter months when vitamin D synthesis is at its lowest.[47]

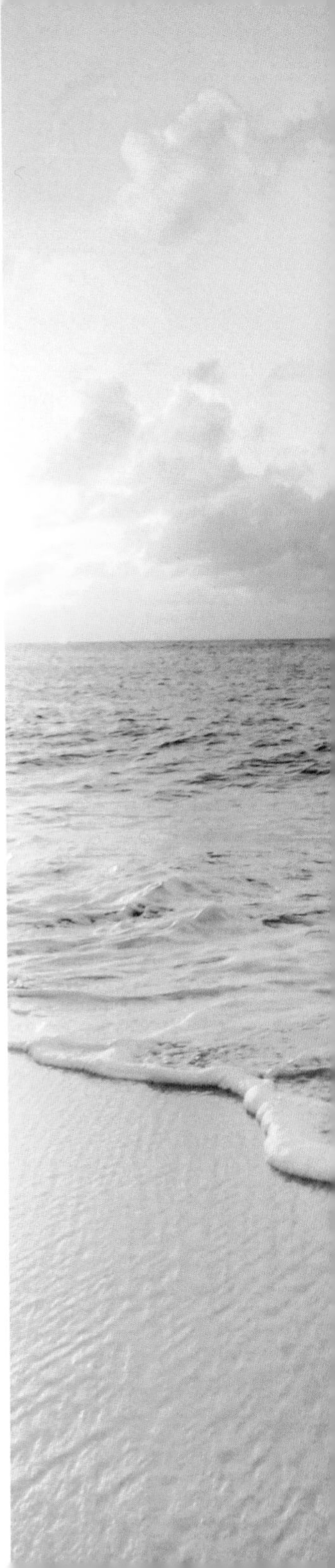

CHAPTER 3

The Mental and Emotional Benefits of the Sea

"If the ocean can calm
itself, so can you.
We are both salt water
mixed with air."

— Nayyirah Waheed

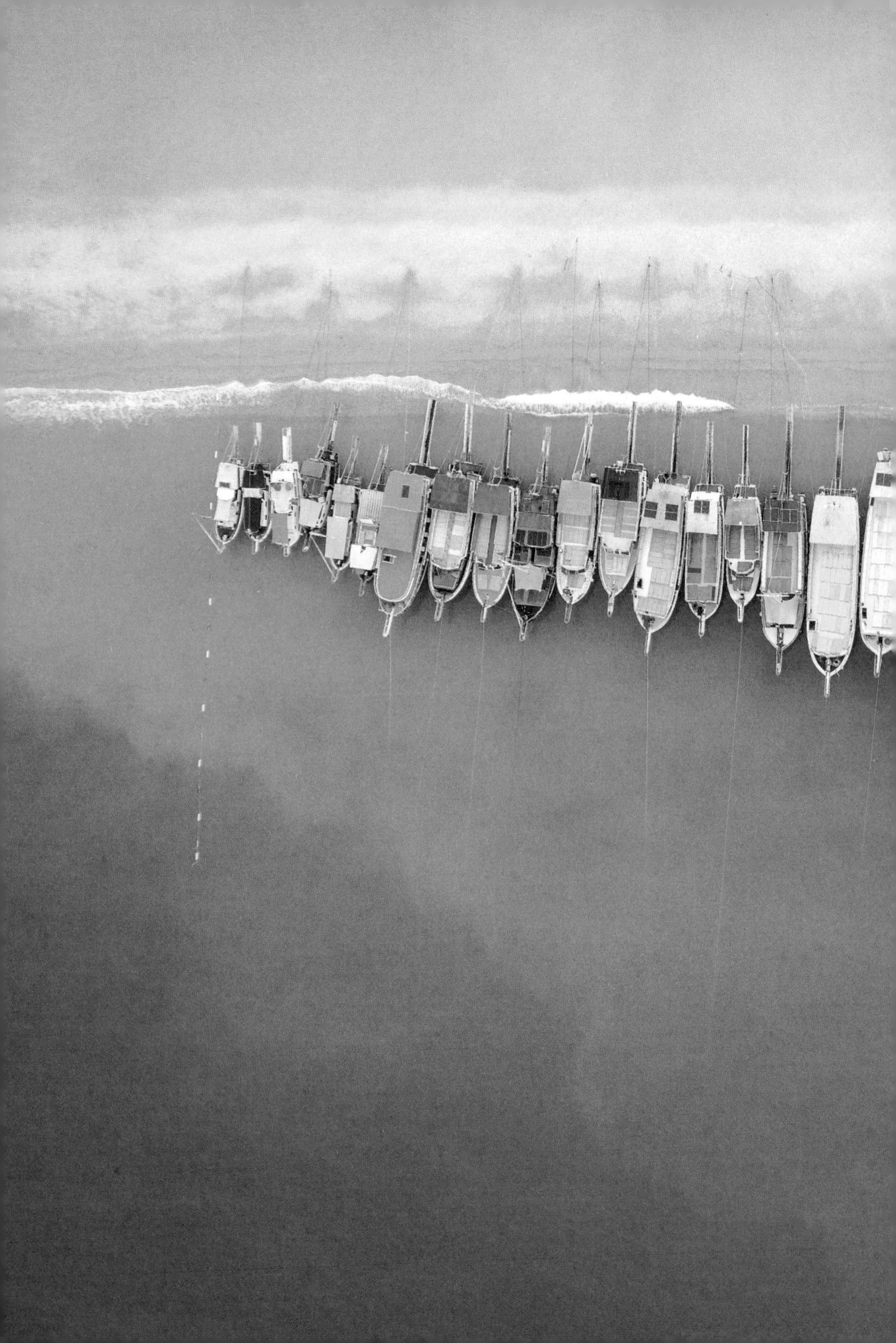

Humans have long had emotional ties with water: water can create meaning and define a location in life, providing an important sense of belonging and attachment.[109, 110] Throughout history, we have used water in religious ceremonies and rituals and may associate certain places, such as sacred wells or the coast, with "healing" experiences.[9]

We still develop emotional attachments to water today and, in particular, with the sea. For some of us, coastal settings are a favourite, everyday place for general recreation and leisure,[111] whereas others may associate certain seaside places with happy memories of childhood holidays or activities we like to pursue. For many people, however, simply seeing the sea can be enough to bring instant feelings of calm and relaxation.

Our physical and mental health are inextricably linked – just as poor physical health can lead to poor mental health, poor mental health can affect our physical health. As such, potentially, one of the main benefits of being by the sea is the way it can calm and rejuvenate the mind, rather than directly heal the body.[7]

There are several theories as to why we feel better being in natural, rather than urban, settings (see pages 31–6). It is likely that we automatically respond in a positive way to living things and landscape features that have helped us survive and thrive throughout our evolutionary past. Water has been found to be a dominant feature of such "restorative" landscapes[25] – viewing water creates strong positive reactions which improve our mood and promote recovery from stress and mental fatigue.[112] So why and how does water have such a powerful effect on us emotionally and psychologically? And, importantly, what evidence is there that being by the sea or, at the very least, viewing the ocean, is particularly beneficial for our emotional health and wellbeing?

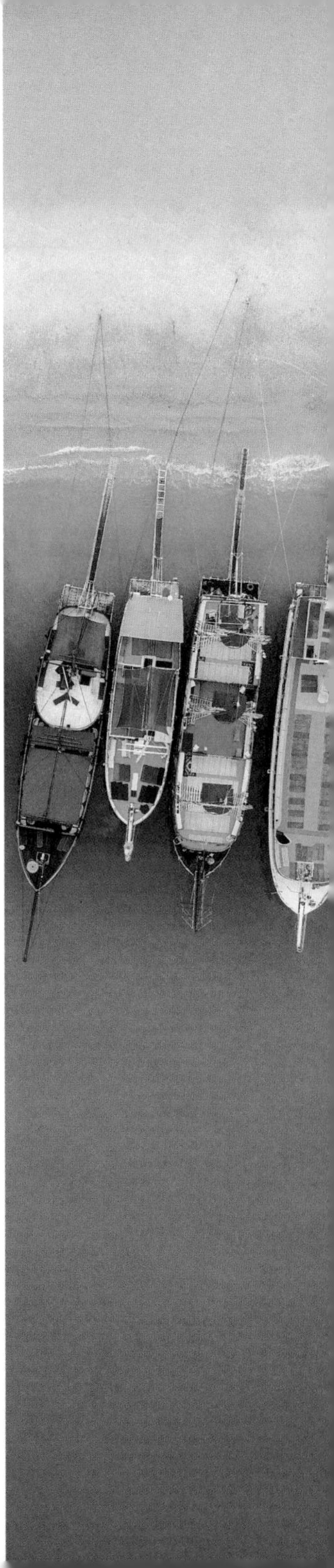

Looking at the Evidence

There are many sources of evidence to support the notion that being by the sea or viewing seascapes is beneficial for our health and wellbeing.

ECONOMICS-BASED RESEARCH

One source of evidence comes from the field of economics, particularly the study of the psychological factors that affect our behaviours and the economic decisions we make. Time and money are two of our most precious resources and there is a substantial amount of evidence from around the world suggesting that people are willing to devote significant amounts of both on being by the sea, whether by living near to the coast or by visiting the seaside for recreation.

Indeed, people are willing to spend a premium to guarantee these coastal experiences – homes with a view of the coast usually cost more than comparable homes without a sea view.[7] And the greater cost associated with a view of the sea will not be lost on anyone who has booked a beach holiday: rooms with that all-important sea view are invariably more expensive than rooms with a view inland.[46]

PSYCHOLOGY-BASED RESEARCH

Exploring how people feel when exposed to different settings and how "restorative" they find these settings can take place either in a laboratory or in "the field" (that is, in a "real" environment). Laboratory studies enable people to experience many different environments without actually moving. For instance, they may rate dozens of photographs of different environments and score each one on several different measures, such as how pleasant the environment looks or how happy the setting makes them feel.

However, the disadvantage is that people are only being asked how they are affected by the visual qualities of a scene, rather than experiencing the real environment with its sounds and smells. Experiencing the "real" environment would seem like the best approach, but it is difficult to collect large amounts of data on specific places and visits, so field experiments tend to use very broad categories (for example, urban versus natural settings). Unfortunately, this fails to establish which features of the landscape (such as water, vegetation, wildlife) are most beneficial to health and wellbeing.[19, 113]

The MENE Survey

One solution is to examine existing data from surveys that have been collected over several years. The Monitoring Engagement with the Natural Environment (MENE) survey started in 2009 and looks at how people in England use the natural environment. Around 45,000 in-depth interviews are conducted annually. Environments are classified into 16 specific types (for example: town park, playing field, woodland, mountain, beach, coast) in three categories: urban green, rural green and coast. Researchers investigated people's feelings about a particular visit to a natural environment made within the last seven days. They asked how "restorative" people thought their experience had been, for example how "calm and relaxed" and how "refreshed and revitalized" they felt.

Of the three categories, people felt more restored when visiting a rural green environment compared to an urban green space. Visits to the coast, however, were more restorative than the other two. Taking a closer look at the 16 specific types, the coast was perceived as more restorative than open countryside but equally restorative as woodlands and upland areas.[112]

A Study of Coastal Residents

Other studies have revealed similar findings. One study explored the coastal experiences that help support and preserve people's personal wellbeing in their everyday lives. The personal activity of 33 residents from two coastal towns in south-west England was tracked for a week, showing where they went, how long they stayed and how active they were. The residents explained why they engaged with different local environments to

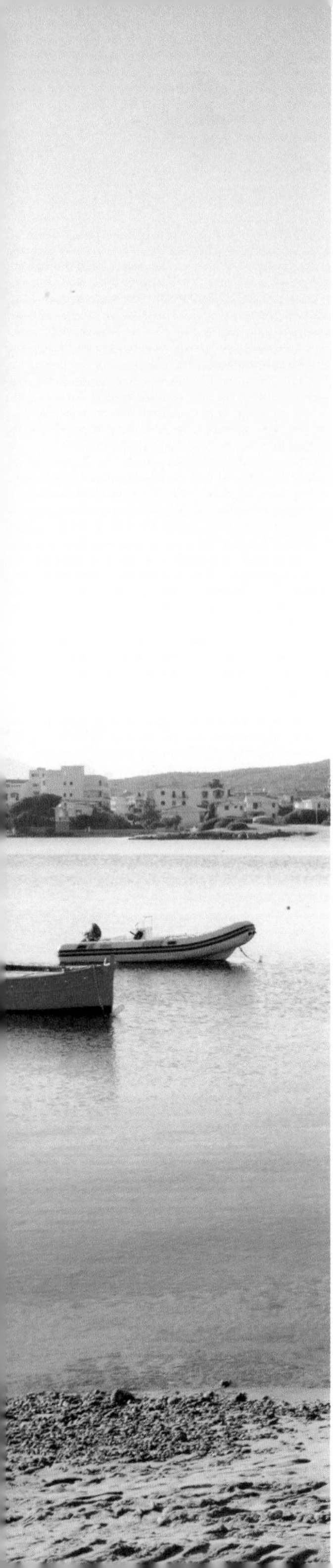

promote and maintain their sense of wellbeing.[9]
This study revealed four main ways in which residents expressed their feelings about the coast:

- **Symbolic** – The sea was "cleansing" and "purifying"; they could get lost in simply watching the sea, and the waves "washed away" their emotions, making them feel calmer; the sea reminded them to occasionally "stop and pause" and not become overwhelmed by life's minutiae, but to take in the bigger picture; they felt "rooted" to the sea and missed the sea when away from home, describing an "itch" to return.

- **Achieving** – The coast was a place where they could fulfil their desire for challenge through a range of activities – such as cycling, walking, kayaking and surfing – allowing them pursue personal, meaningful goals; unlike a gym, the coast was a pleasurable environment which also had cognitive and emotional benefits. Activities like surfing and sailing, especially in challenging weather conditions, may be physically uncomfortable but can offer a moment of highly intense happiness and fulfilment, contributing to feelings of competence, purpose and achievement.

- **Immersive** – People often engaged in activities like fishing or simply staring out to sea that required little concentration and enabled them to open themselves up to the multisensory experiences offered by the coast, creating the mental space required to reflect and gain a sense of perspective. Different environmental conditions can influence how we feel and have a dramatic effect on our experiences: fine weather and gently lapping waves may be soothing, while watching stormy seas and being exposed to wind and rain can feel more invigorating, giving us a greater sense of "being alive". Watching the waves break was mentioned as being especially relaxing: the repetitive nature of the breaking waves can be quite hypnotic and helpful when dealing with stress. This kind of repetitive, non-threatening motion – sometimes described as Heraclitean motion – can be endlessly fascinating and extremely relaxing.

- **Social** – Local coastal spaces could provide an opportunity for people to find friendly conversation, to engage in family leisure and wellbeing, or connect to others through shared experiences and hobbies; they could bring back happy childhood memories and enable parents to create new memories with their own children. The beach seems a particularly good location for "family bonding" as it seems to meet the needs of both children and adults.

Comparing Coastal Residents with Those Living Inland

Two UK-based studies have compared the self-reported health of people living by the coast with those who live further inland, or who did not have a sea view.

The first study used the 2001 census data from England, which included a question asking people to rate their health over the last 12 months as "good", "fairly good" or "not good". The researchers found that the closer to the sea a person lived, the more likely they were to report good health. Importantly, the positive health benefits appeared to be greater for those from more socio-economically deprived communities, suggesting that living by the coast may lessen some of the negative health effects of poverty and deprivation. Similar results have been found in green space settings.[114]

Although this study gives an interesting insight into the relationship between distance from the sea and reported good health, is it only a snapshot in time: presenting data from one census year does not account for how people's health changes over time. Maybe their good health was down to the fact that they were healthy and wealthy enough to move to a more desirable area, such as the coast?

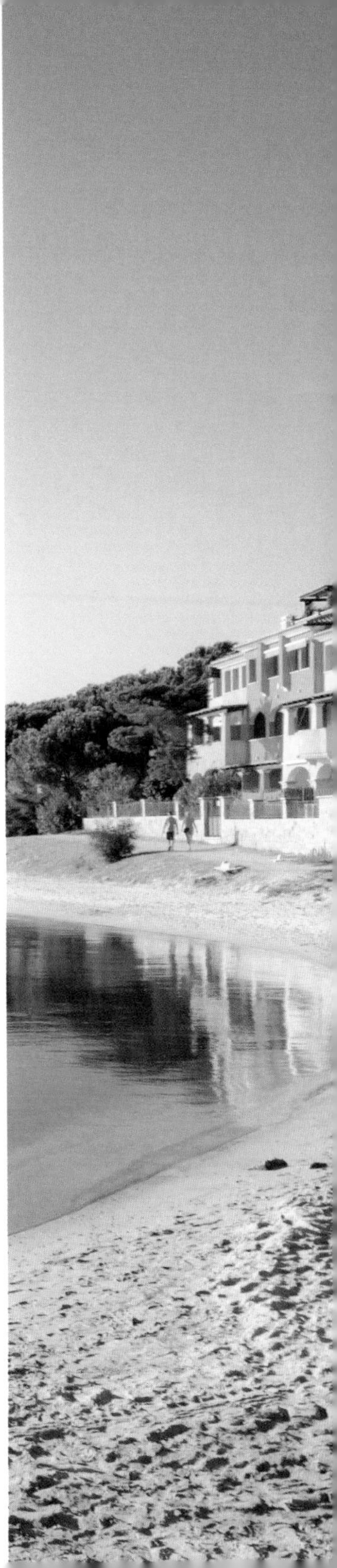

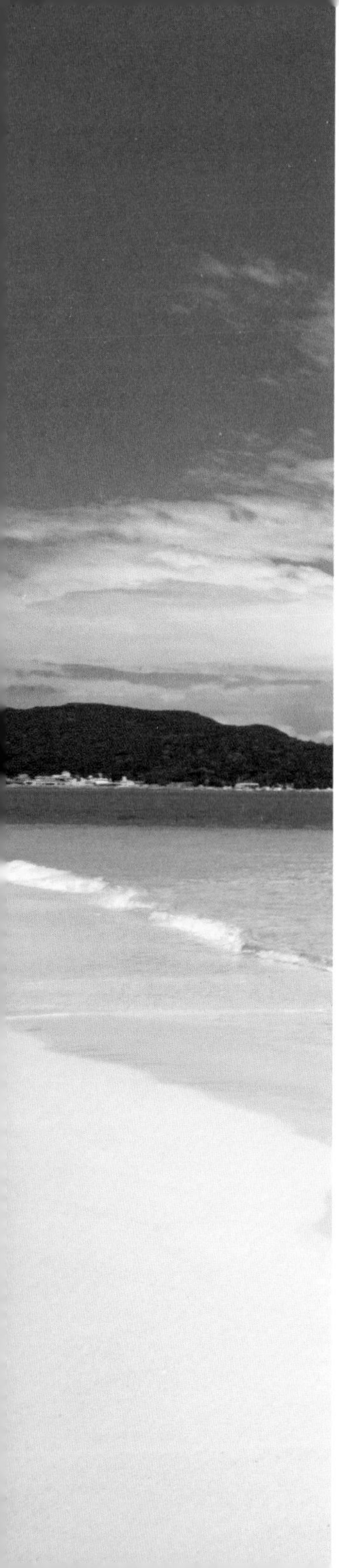

A further study was conducted to compare people's overall self-reported health when they lived in one particular location, compared to when living in other locations.[112] It revealed that individuals reported better general health and mental health in the years that they lived close to the sea. It also appeared that the benefits of living by the sea were more strongly associated with a reduction in negative effects (such as mental distress), than an increase in positive effects (such as feelings of wellbeing). Considering evidence from the studies already mentioned, this seems to make sense: other research has found that being by the sea may help reduce stress, encourage physical activity and foster positive social interactions, all of which have been associated with positive health benefits.

A Japanese Study

Similar results have been found in Japan. One study compared responses from residents of two residential areas in Japan: one with and one without an ocean view.[115] Residents completed a questionnaire that asked them to report how much they agreed or disagreed with statements about the following things:

- **The passage of time** – for example, "You can forget how time flies."
- **Magnitude and awe** – for example, "You can feel the magnitude and richness of nature."
- **Peace of mind** – for example, "You can feel the tranquillity."
- **Charm and longing** – for example, "You can feel longing and hope."
- **Threat** – for example, "You can feel uncomfortable."

The researchers found that people who live near the sea showed higher positive psychological effects for passage of time, magnitude and awe, peace of mind, and charm and longing, but lower negative effects for threat, when compared to those residents who lived inland. They also found that the positive effects of coastal settings were greater for females than males. This is perhaps because, in Japanese culture, there are many full-time "housewives" and spending more time at home gave them more time to look at the sea, and avoid a stressful office environment.

Residents of all ages felt more positive psychological benefits if they lived by the sea, rather than inland, but the positive effects were strongest for elderly residents, perhaps because they too spend more time at home exposed to the positive effects of the sea. Overall, the study concluded that living by the sea makes residents experience more positive emotions, such as a sense of peace and calm, and promotes general wellbeing.

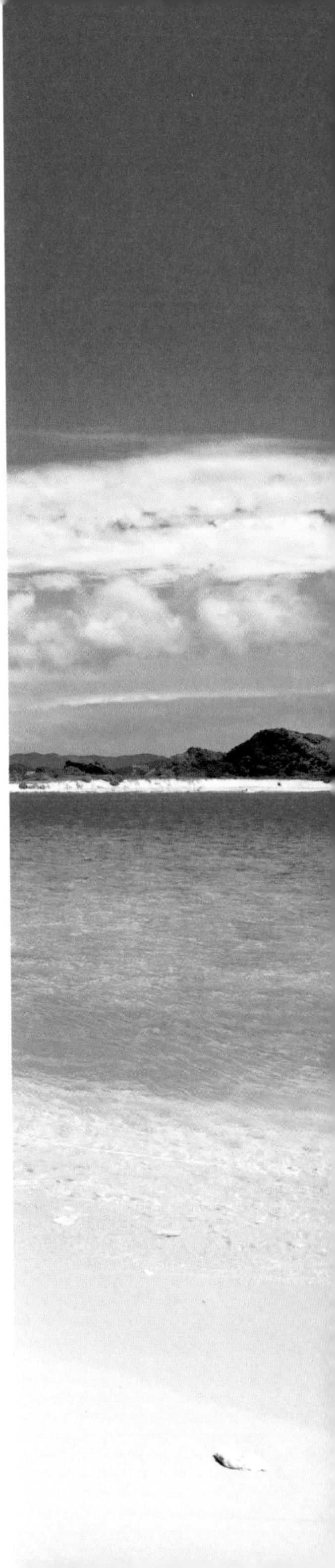

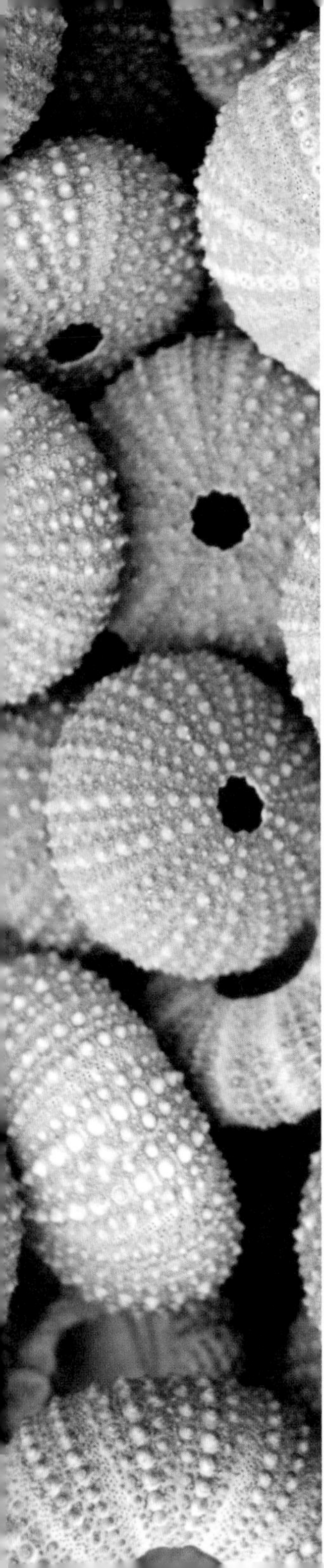

The Properties of Water

Spending time in and around the sea is a rich experience that engages all five senses. The sight of the blue sea, the sound of breaking waves, the smell of the ocean, the taste of salt on your lips, the feeling of warm sand between your toes or the cool water all around you are all sensory experiences that create positive feelings and emotions and enhance our wellbeing. Perhaps some of the properties of water itself contribute to these feelings.

THE LOOK OF THE SEA

Colour is an important part of our visual experience, influencing many of our behaviours, such as which car to buy or what clothes to wear.[116] The colour most positively associated with water is blue. We love seeing the blue waters of the ocean – from the lightest aquamarine of the shallow waters to the deepest sapphire blue of the ocean depths. Many people cite blue as their favourite colour. Indeed, a worldwide survey spanning ten countries, across four continents, revealed that blue is the most popular colour, even in places like China, where certain colours – such as red, yellow and green – are regarded as lucky or auspicious.

Psychologists and marketers have found that people associate the colour blue with qualities such as credibility, openness, trust, depth and wisdom.[117] Commonly the colour blue is associated with feelings of calmness or serenity; some people paint rooms in their home blue to create a peaceful and tranquil environment.[118] Although the colour blue can have some less positive associations, such as coldness and "feeling blue" (sad), overall, blue appeals to people of all ages and is often the favourite colour of both men and women.[119]

Perhaps one reason why we prefer images of the coast, and other aquatic settings, is our strong preference for the colour blue. Seeking to understand a little more about how favourite colours affect people's preferences for different landscapes, researchers from the UK compared people's responses to images of three environments (urban, rural/green, aquatic) taken in black and white, rather than colour. They found that people still preferred images of aquatic environments to images of rural/green and urban scenes, even when viewing those images in monochrome. This suggests that any preference for the colour blue may relate more to our evolutionary history than simply a preference for the colour. Perhaps we are drawn to the colour blue as it signifies a potential source of fresh water and food, and hence life.[120]

Patterns created by the way water reflects light as it moves capture people's attention and can be fascinating. One type of these – fractal patterns – are particularly interesting as it has been suggested that some of the psychological and physiological benefits of viewing nature can be explained by nature's fractal properties.[121] Fractals (a term first used by mathematician Benoît Mandelbrot in 1975) occur when a similar pattern repeats itself as it gets larger or smaller.[122] Fractal patterns can either be "exact", whereby the pattern repeats itself exactly at different scales, or "statistical", a more random fractal pattern found in nature.[121] Think of the way a tree trunk divides into increasingly smaller branches and eventually into twigs – this is an example of a natural (statistical) fractal pattern.

There are many such fascinating patterns in nature: the fronds of a fern, a snail's shell, a river delta and Romanesco broccoli. Fractal patterns can also be found on the coast – ocean waves, clouds and even the coastline itself contain natural fractal patterns that people find captivating. Studies comparing people's responses to the two different types of fractal patterns suggest that the type found in nature is important for inducing "alpha responses" in the brain, indicative of a wakeful, relaxed state.[121]

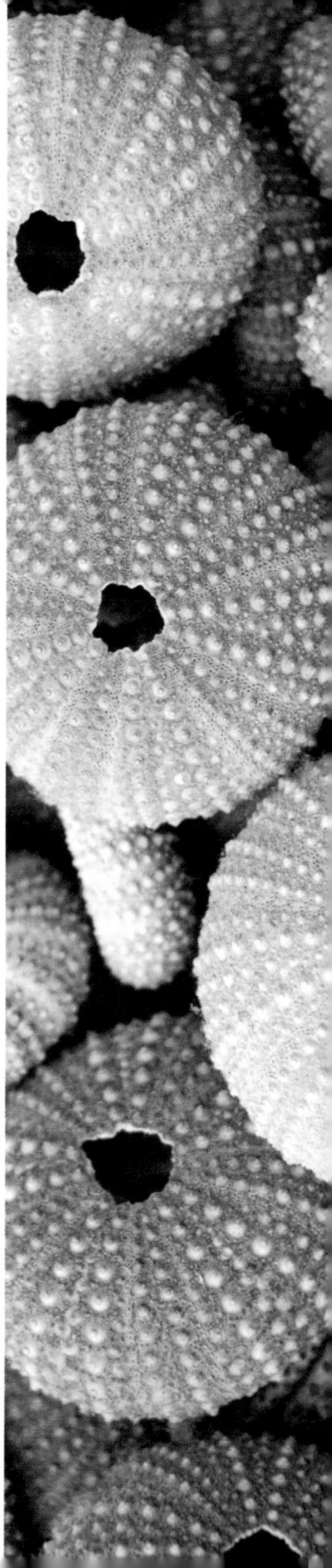

THE SOUND OF THE SEA

The sound of water is also extremely restorative and can generating feelings of relaxation.[123] Many relaxation aids, such as CDs and apps, deliberately feature water sounds, for example breaking waves on a beach, as they are thought to help us relax and de-stress.

For some people, the sounds, smells and touch of the sea may be especially valuable. Studies conducted with people with impaired sight have highlighted the importance of the auditory, olfactory and tactile aspects of a coastal visit. While they may not be able to appreciate the colour of the sea or the patterns on the water, it is still possible to benefit from the sea's other relaxing and invigorating qualities.

THE TOUCH, TASTE AND SMELL OF THE SEA

The senses can be immersed in the seascape by listening to the waves, smelling the seaweed and feeling the sand.[70] Also, water can also be, quite literally, immersive. Swimming and bathing in water creates an altogether different way to experience the natural environment that is not possible on land.[124] Research using flotation tanks has found that immersion in water can be beneficial for many psychological and physiological problems – decreasing stress, anxiety, depression and perceived pain, and increasing optimism and quality of sleep (see page 136).[125]

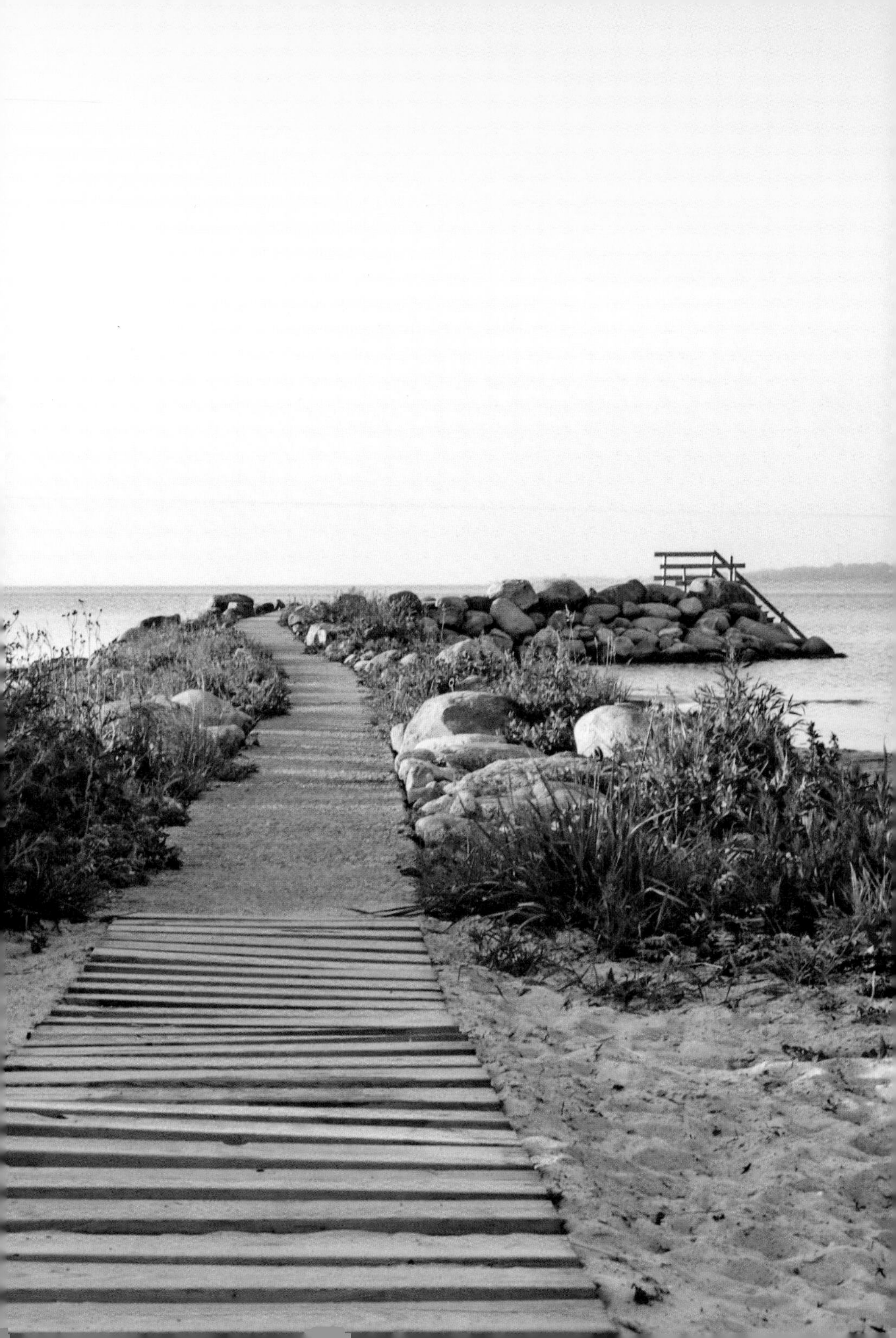

The Effects of Marine Life on Health and Wellbeing

People not only enjoy the sights, smells and sounds of the sea, but also appreciate the chance to experience the flora and fauna. Dolphins, seals, whales, basking sharks and sea birds are all species people hope to catch a glimpse of around the coast. Easier to spot are the coastal plants and wildflowers that adorn the rocky shores, cliff tops, beaches, dunes and estuaries. It goes without saying that family days spent looking for crabs and small fishes amid the rock pool seaweeds, or beachcombing for empty shells, can create their own special memories.

While seeing some of the remarkable plants and animals that inhabit our coastline can have a profound effect on our day, little research has been carried out in the actual marine environment itself: most studies have been conducted using indirect experiences of marine life such as viewing photographs in a laboratory setting. Nevertheless, these studies provide some evidence of the beneficial effects that seeing marine life can have on our health and wellbeing.

One such study used photographs and video clips of the flora and fauna found along the UK coast to explore how different numbers and types of marine species made people feel. The study found that coastal scenes containing greater numbers of plants and animals made people feel better and more restored than settings with less marine life. Furthermore, an animal's behaviour also influenced how people felt. For instance, watching animals engage in interesting behaviours – gannets diving for food, seals playing in the surf – improved people's mood more than watching the same animals doing less interesting things, such as gannets nesting on a cliff or seals sleeping on the beach.[126]

STUDIES IN AQUARIUMS

Studies in public aquariums have found similar findings. In one study, people's behavioural, psychological and physiological responses to three different levels of marine life in a large public aquarium exhibit were investigated. The study ran during three stages of restocking: first, when the exhibit was unstocked and contained only water and artificial seaweed; a second time when it was partially stocked with the first newly quarantined fish and crustaceans; and a final time when the exhibit was fully stocked.[127]

Observations revealed that aquarium visitors tended to spend longer in front of the exhibit when it was fully stocked. It is likely that the visitors found the greater level of marine life more fascinating to watch. This effortless, "soft" fascination would have created an opportunity to forget about their daily routines and concerns, and thus promoted psychological restoration.

During the second part of the study, participants answered five evaluation questions about their experiences.

- Evaluations were actually positive in all three stocking conditions: participants found watching the exhibit made them feel better and was enjoyable and interesting.
- People's responses to the five evaluation questions, however, were significantly more positive for the partially and fully stocked exhibit than the unstocked exhibit.
- For two evaluation statements, participants rated the fully stocked exhibit significantly higher than the partially stocked phase.
- The different levels of marine life also affected mood: people generally became calmer and more positive the longer they spent viewing the exhibit.
- Interestingly, however, at the higher level of marine life people felt less calm, most likely because the greater level of marine life was more interesting to watch.
- There were significant drops in heart rate during all stages of restocking but the drops in heart rate were significantly greater when the exhibit contained any marine life.

Do We Prefer Some Creatures to Others?

Although the above study investigated people's reactions to different amounts of marine life in one specific exhibit, public aquariums usually display a variety of large and small tropical and temperate exhibits. Exhibits may house a single interesting specimen (such as a giant Pacific octopus, *Enteroctopus dofleini*), a mixed community of different fish from a specific habitat, or a large number of the same species (such as a shoal of Northern anchovies, *Engraulis mordax*). Some exhibits feature typically

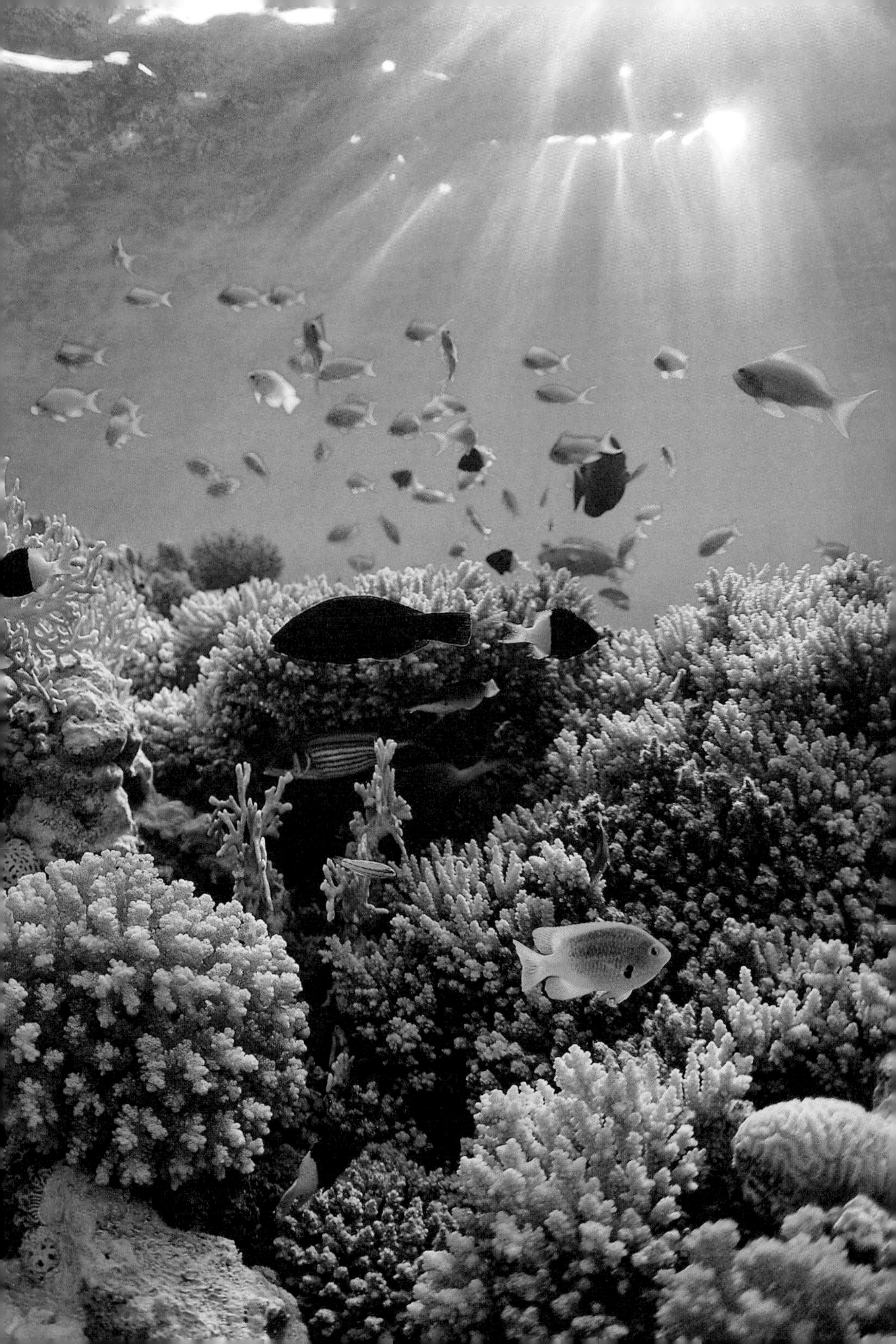

charismatic species, such as seahorses,[128] whereas other exhibits may contain anecdotally less appealing animals, such as crabs.[129,130]

Anecdotal observations of public aquarium visitors suggest that many have preferences for particular animals and respond in emotionally different ways to different exhibits.

Therefore another study investigated the influence of exhibit type on people's health and wellbeing, using a set of 40 photographs of public aquarium exhibits, categorized by broad climatic region (such as temperate or tropical), and by whether they contained high or low numbers of species and individuals.[131] Participants rated all the photographs on four measures, including "how pleasant" they found the image, how the image "made them feel" and "how restorative" they perceived the image to be.

- Participants tended to rate the highly colourful tropical exhibits more favourably than the less vibrant temperate exhibits, potentially supporting previous studies in which people have expressed a preference for plant arrays containing greater, rather than fewer, brightly coloured flowers.[132]
- Exhibits containing a high abundance of animals, a variety of species, and charismatic animals were also usually preferred to exhibits that contained fewer animals or species, or "less interesting" animals.
- People also rated images of schooling fish relatively highly. A school of fish differs from a shoal of fish in that a school usually contains similarly sized and aged fish of the same species moving together in a tight group. Schooling fish, such as anchovies and sardines, swim at the same speed and in the same direction as each other and this coordinated movement can result in some intricate formations and manoeuvres, including "bait balls", a strategy employed when threatened by predators. It is possible that people rated these images quite highly because the bait ball movement is an example of repetitive and hypnotic Heraclitean motion (see pages 68–9).

These studies indicate that, when it comes to our emotions, all animals are not created equal – we prefer some animals to others and some animals can have an especially strong effect on our emotions. Unlike rocks, trees and plants, we feel more connected to animals as we can relate to some of the struggles they face to survive. Like us they battle against the weather, are constantly aware of threats such as predators, need to find food for themselves and/or their families, and can mourn the loss of a family or community member.[133]

STUDIES IN NATURE

One study has explored people's feelings after wildlife encounters in the real marine environment and provides an intriguing insight into how these wildlife encounters can positively impact on a person's wellbeing. Participants on a whale- and bird-watching excursion were interviewed about their experiences and many struggled to adequately express their feelings about these encounters. One participant on a whale-watching trip commented "...there are no words to describe what the whales were like. It is sort of a feeling that you have...a...real sense of wellbeing and positive rush."[133]

- The wildlife excursions lifted the spirits, facilitated contemplation and provided a time to "stand and stare".
- They elicited feelings of deep joy and happiness.
- The participants expressed a sense of awe and wonder for nature's beauty and design.
- They felt an awakening of their senses and an altered sense of time – they experienced a state of "flow".

Experiencing Flow

Chances are, "flow" is something that many of us will have experienced at some point in our lives. It occurs when we have an "optimal" experience; an experience during which we feel a sense of exhilaration and a deep sense of enjoyment. We tend to cherish these experiences for a long time and they stand out as landmarks in our lives. These experiences are usually not passive or relaxing times, but times when we push our body or mind to its limits in a voluntary effort, or achieve something that is deemed difficult or worthwhile. We are so engaged in an activity that is so enjoyable that nothing else matters: we may feel an altered state of time while we are "in the zone".[134]

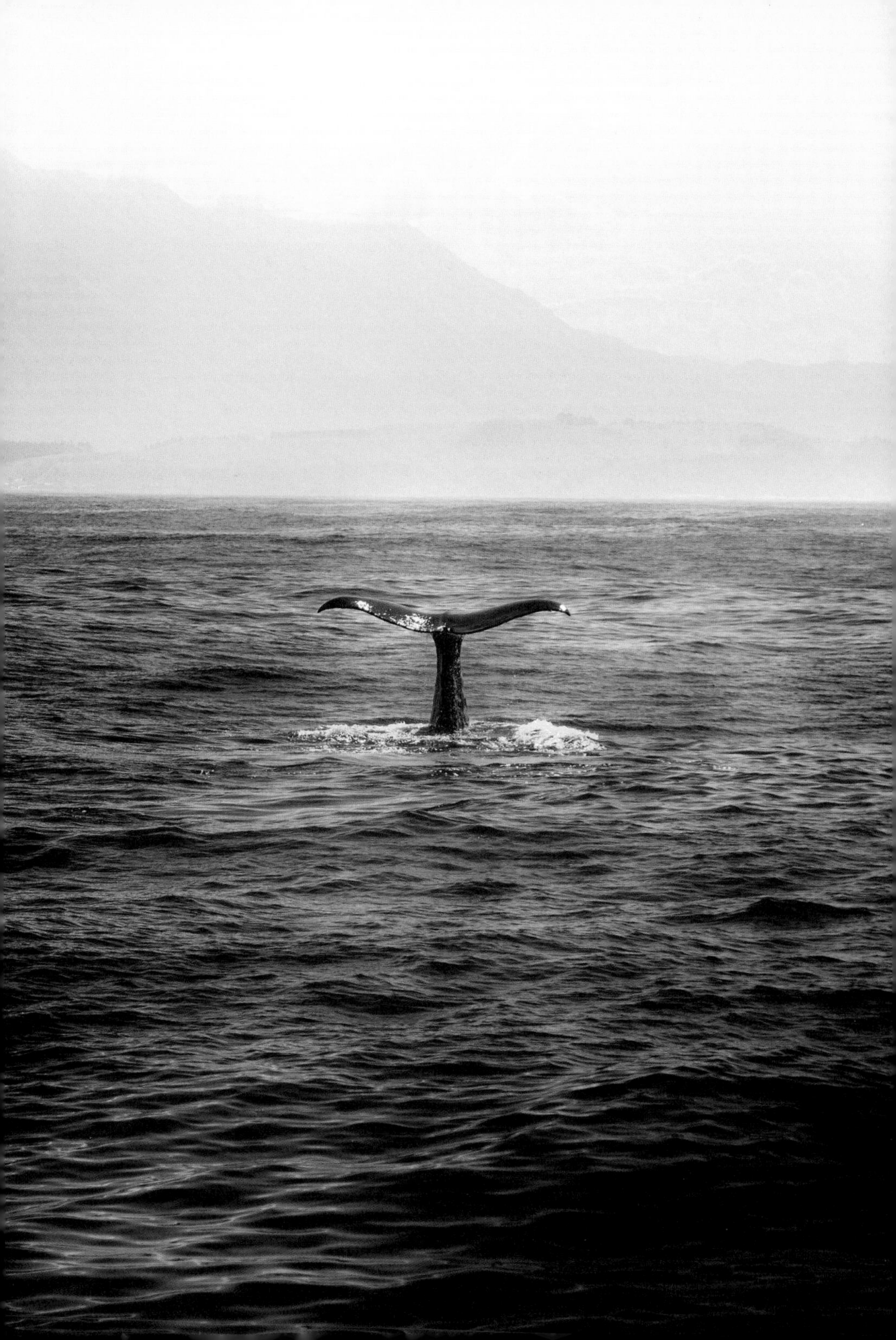

ANIMAL-ASSISTED THERAPY

Whales and dolphins are incredibly "charismatic" as they exhibit several characteristics we find appealing, so people are especially keen to experience these animals. People refer to dolphins as intelligent, beautiful, serene and playful,[130] and it is these characteristics that have doubtless made them popular for the treatment of illness and developmental disabilities.

Dolphin-assisted therapy (DAT) provides participants with the opportunity to swim or interact with live captive dolphins.[135] There are numerous facilities around the world – including in the Unites States, Japan, China, Russia and Mexico – that provide this form of therapy. Proponents of DAT believe that these interactions can help people with clinical disorders and diseases – such as autism, epilepsy, multiple sclerosis, depression and cancer – by increasing stimulation, improving memory and motor skills, accelerating the healing of disease, and increasing wellbeing. However, there isn't much robust scientific evidence on the effectiveness of DAT, and some believe that the best that can be realistically suggested is that any perceived benefits originate from the sheer pleasure of swimming with these wonderful animals.[135]

Dolphins are one of the few aquatic animals that are used in animal-assisted therapy (AAT), as most treatments involve land-based animals such as dogs.[136] However, captive grey or harbour seals have been the subject of a recent case study (Project Seal to Heal) investigating whether interacting with seals could help a war veteran with PTSD-like symptoms. The study found that, overall, participation in Project Seal to Heal resulted in a clinically significant reduction in PTSD-like symptoms for the veteran who completed the programme.[137]

Viewing the animals within public aquarium exhibits has also been found to benefit human health and wellbeing (see pages 76–7)[127] and this could be viewed as an animal-assisted therapy. Indeed, even keeping a small fish tank at home has been found to be beneficial to health. In a survey of 100 home aquarium owners:

- 94 per cent of respondents felt that they benefitted from their aquarium.
- Around 70 per cent of respondents stated that they found watching their fish calming, relaxing and helpful in reducing stress and anxiety levels.
- A small number of male respondents mentioned that their doctors had suggested owning a home aquarium to help lower their blood pressure.[138]

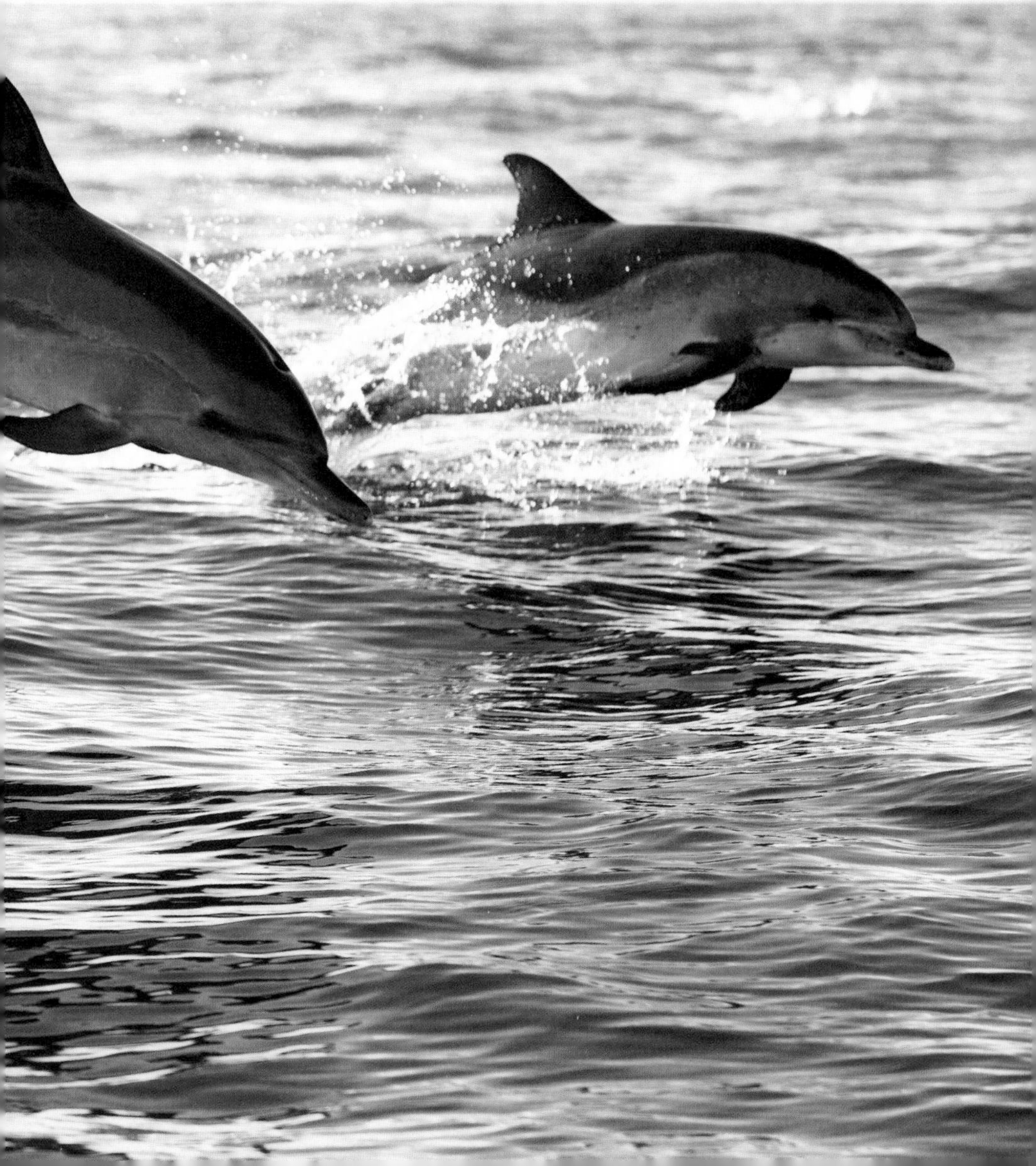

Family Time

In a study looking at how families spent time at the beach, researchers found that the whole family felt the psychological benefits of experiencing fun, happiness and enjoyment. Both children and adults also felt that the beach was a relaxing and restorative location: the sound of the waves and the beauty of the setting all contributed to helping them to feel calm and less stressed.[6]

Spending time at the beach was also found to benefit social interactions. Children felt that their families spent more time interacting with them when at the beach compared with other settings. A range of important skills may be passed from adults to children during these times: instruction on learning to swim or surf, how to respect rock pool habitats by taking care to return rocks to their original positions, and not startling or chasing fish.

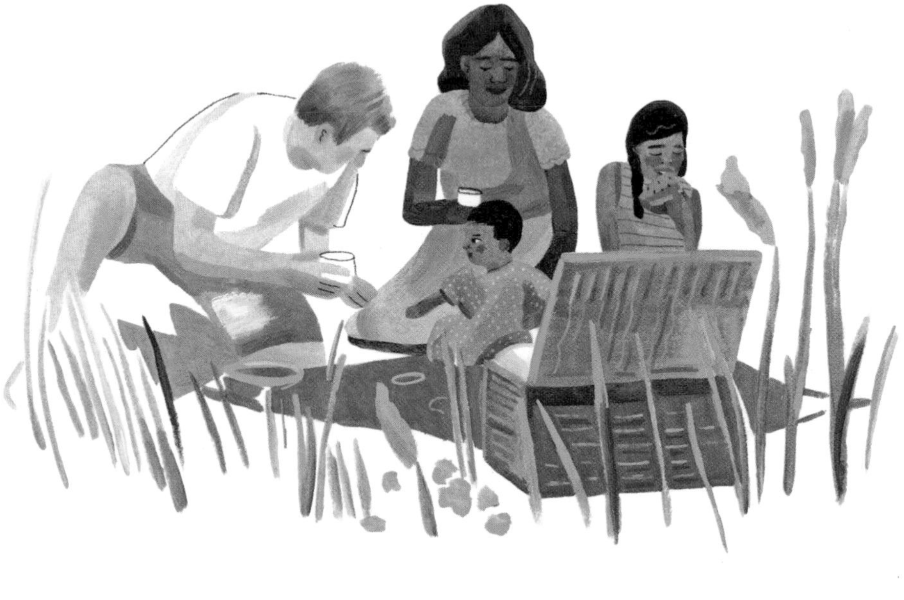

THE IMPORTANCE OF PLAY

The beach is also a wonderful location for children to play on their own (albeit under a distant and watchful eye). The beach offers many opportunities for children to explore for themselves, doing whatever they feel like doing – peering in caves, looking in rock pools and climbing on rocks. Play is essential to a child's development as it contributes to cognitive, social, physical and emotional wellbeing.[139]

Undirected play – without parents or other adults present – is particularly important as it gives children a sense of freedom and control. It encourages creativity, exploration and self-learning – including learning from their mistakes. Undirected play allows children to make new friends, learn to work in groups, to share, to resolve conflicts, to negotiate and express themselves.[139] They get to practice important decision-making skills, enabling them to decide what they want to do and learn what things they like and dislike. Playing in natural environments allows children to develop an awareness of their surroundings and gain an appreciation of nature.

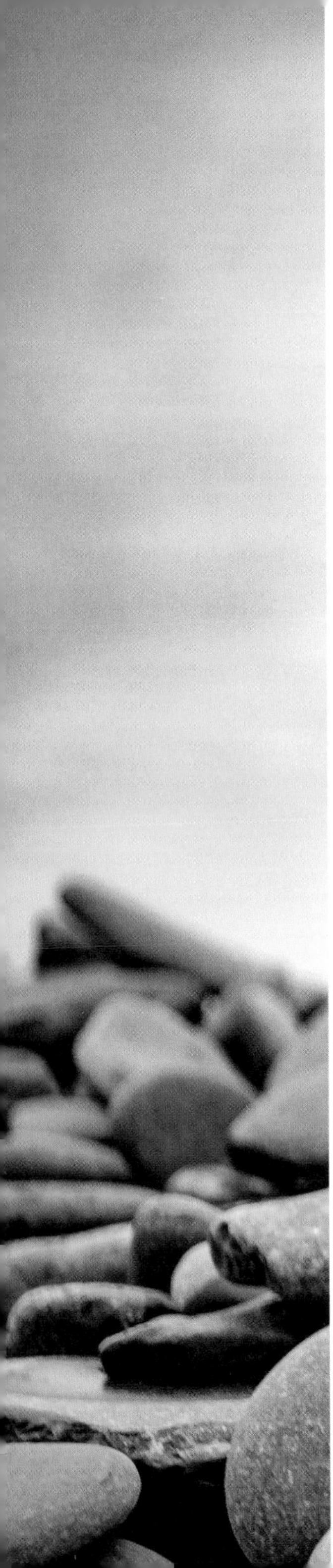

Increasing Access to the Sea

Our own intuitive reactions – increasingly supported by scientific studies – suggest that we feel better when we are by the sea and it is good for our physical and mental health and wellbeing. Unfortunately, not everyone is able or willing to spend time at the sea and benefit from this precious natural resource. Some of the reasons may relate to access issues, such as reduced physical mobility or ill health, poor local infrastructure (for example insufficient public transport or inadequately maintained coastal paths), financial constraints, or simply having too little free time.

Access may also be limited by a person's psychological abilities, such as lack of confidence, cognitive problems or psychological disorders (for example agoraphobia). Other factors deterring people from visiting blue space environments could include perceptions of poor water quality or the presence of unsightly litter or other types of pollution.[140, 141]

OVERCOMING BARRIERS TO ACCESS

People from the most socio-economically deprived areas, as well as women and the elderly, are the most likely to benefit from the restorative effects of the sea so it is important to encourage all demographic groups within society to visit the coast.

There are various ways that that this can be achieved. Better planning and investment in the marine environment (and related infrastructure and amenities) could help encourage people to spend more time by the coast. Access issues may be costly to rectify in some instances – especially if large-scale changes are needed or they are in especially difficult-to-reach areas – but small-scale changes, often referred to as "urban acupuncture" (see page 89), could prove relatively effective.

To improve engagement with the marine environment and its health-giving properties, it is important that it is perceived as being welcoming: it should have good water quality, be free of litter, feel safe, have well-maintained paths and facilities, and be accessible to all. Although improvements to coastal sites require an investment of valuable time and money, local authorities may consider that it is worth the investment if, ultimately, improving access to and engagement with the marine environment positively benefits the health and wellbeing of the local population.

Any increased engagement with the coast should be carefully managed and monitored. Marine ecosystems can be very fragile: poor marine planning, inappropriate industrial and tourism development, littering, pollution and habitat damage and loss are just some of the pressures the marine environment faces. Therefore, while policy makers may wish to improve access and environmental quality with the aim of promoting public health and wellbeing, care must be taken to ensure that this is properly managed in the face of potentially increased visitor numbers and the associated pressures.[3, 82, 112]

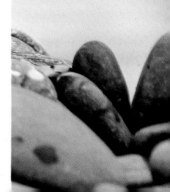

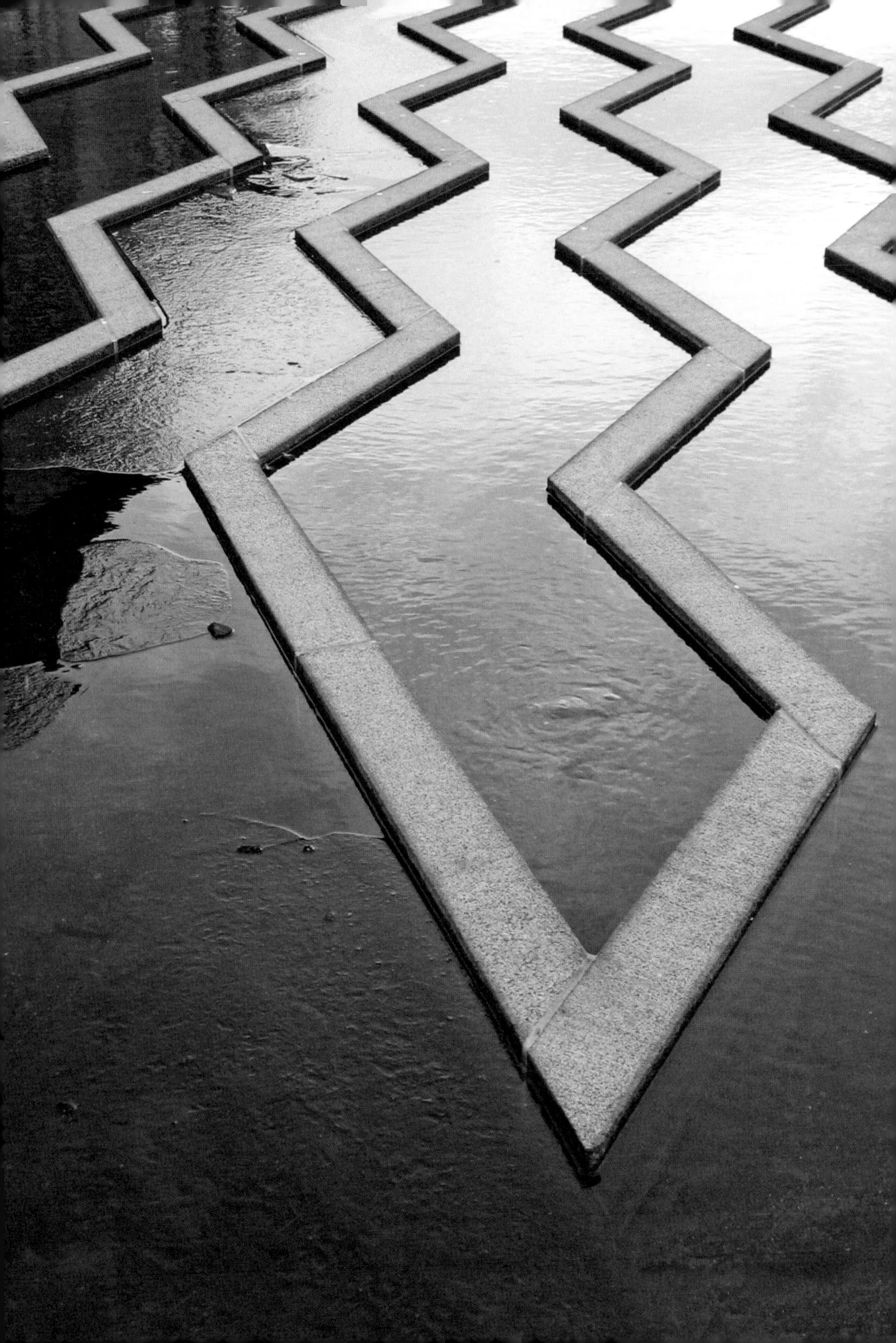

Urban Acupuncture

Urban acupuncture is a technique that can relieve stress and improve the wellbeing of city residents. Developed by Finnish architect and professor Marco Casagrande, urban acupuncture combines Chinese acupuncture with Western urban design theory. Just as Chinese acupuncture uses fine needles to improve the health and wellbeing of the whole person, urban acupuncture uses small-scale interventions at sites that are underused, inaccessible or perceived as negative in some way, to provide disproportionately large positive impacts on the use or enjoyment of those places by its local population.[142, 143]

In the UK, the BlueHealth project (a multi-country, European project) is undertaking an urban acupuncture intervention at a neglected inner-city beach in Plymouth. The project aims to look at the health and wellbeing benefits – for the local community and visitors – that result from improving and regenerating the site: the beach will be cleaned, slipway access will be improved, overgrown vegetation will be controlled, existing children's play equipment will be upgraded, and the site will be landscaped to include seating and a new open-air amphitheatre. These improvements aim to increase engagement with the beach, as well as encourage greater social interaction among residents and visitors, all factors that could improve health and wellbeing.

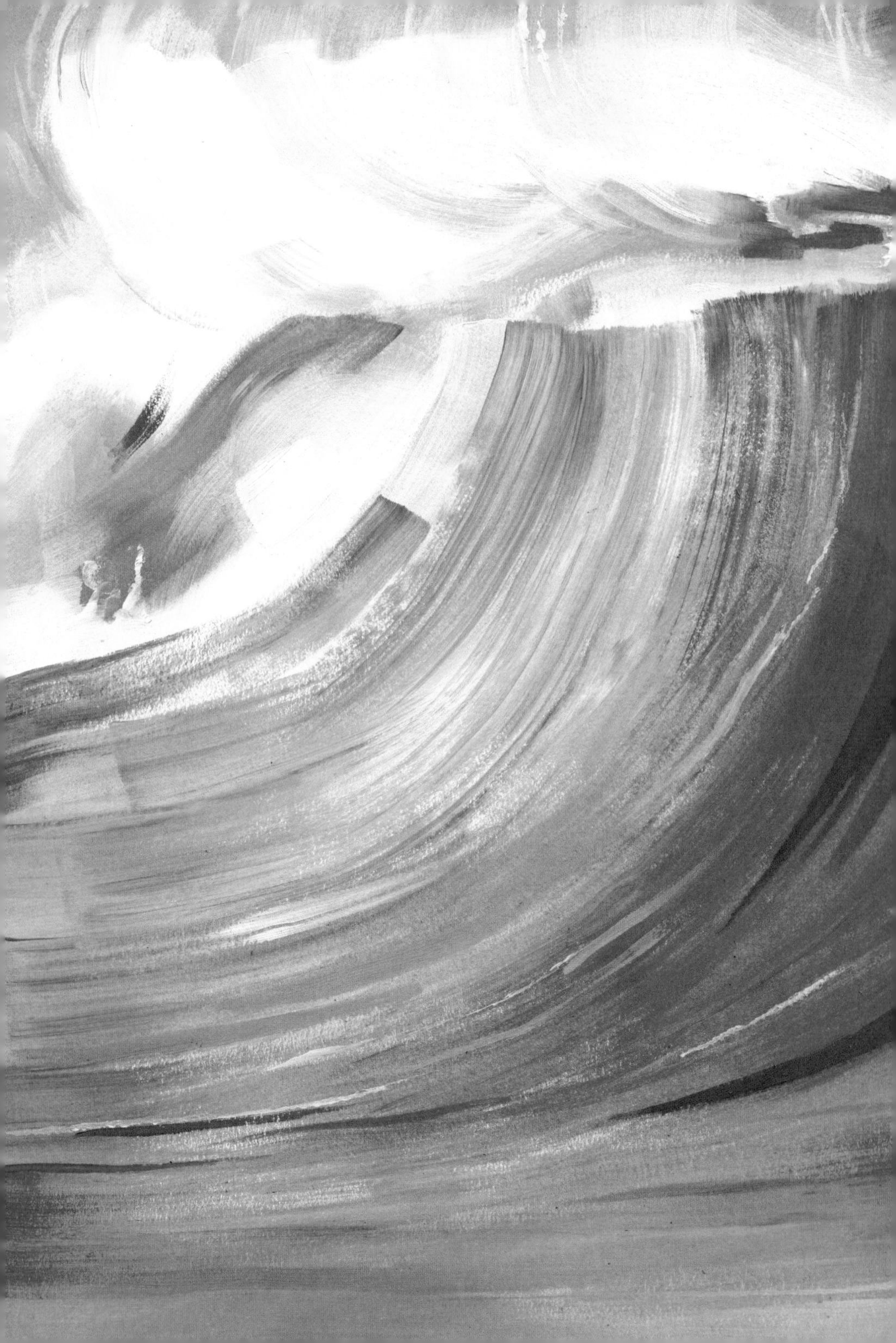

CHAPTER 4

Enhancing the Benefits

"The three great elemental
sounds in nature are the
sound of rain, the sound of
wind in a primeval wood,
and the sound of outer
ocean on a beach.
I have heard them all, and
of the three elemental
voices, that of ocean
is the most awesome,
beautiful and varied."

— Henry Beston

Being immersed in a coastal environment can have positive effects on our wellbeing in so many different ways, so how can we make the most of a trip to the sea to gain as many of those benefits as possible? There are a number of ways to take full advantage and enhance the benefits of the sea and its surroundings.

EXPOSURE TO THE SUN

Spending time near a giant body of water which reflects the sun's rays will allow your body to make plenty of vitamin D, vital for maintaining healthy bones and teeth, promoting digestive health, improving immunity and mental wellbeing and protecting against certain forms of cancer (see pages 60–1). Unfortunately, we can only make vitamin D when our skin is exposed to the sun, not when we are covered up or wearing sunscreen.

If you are out and about in the middle of the day and the sky is clear, be sure to apply sunscreen to prevent burning. At other times, though, allow your skin to get some exposure to the sun before you cover up.

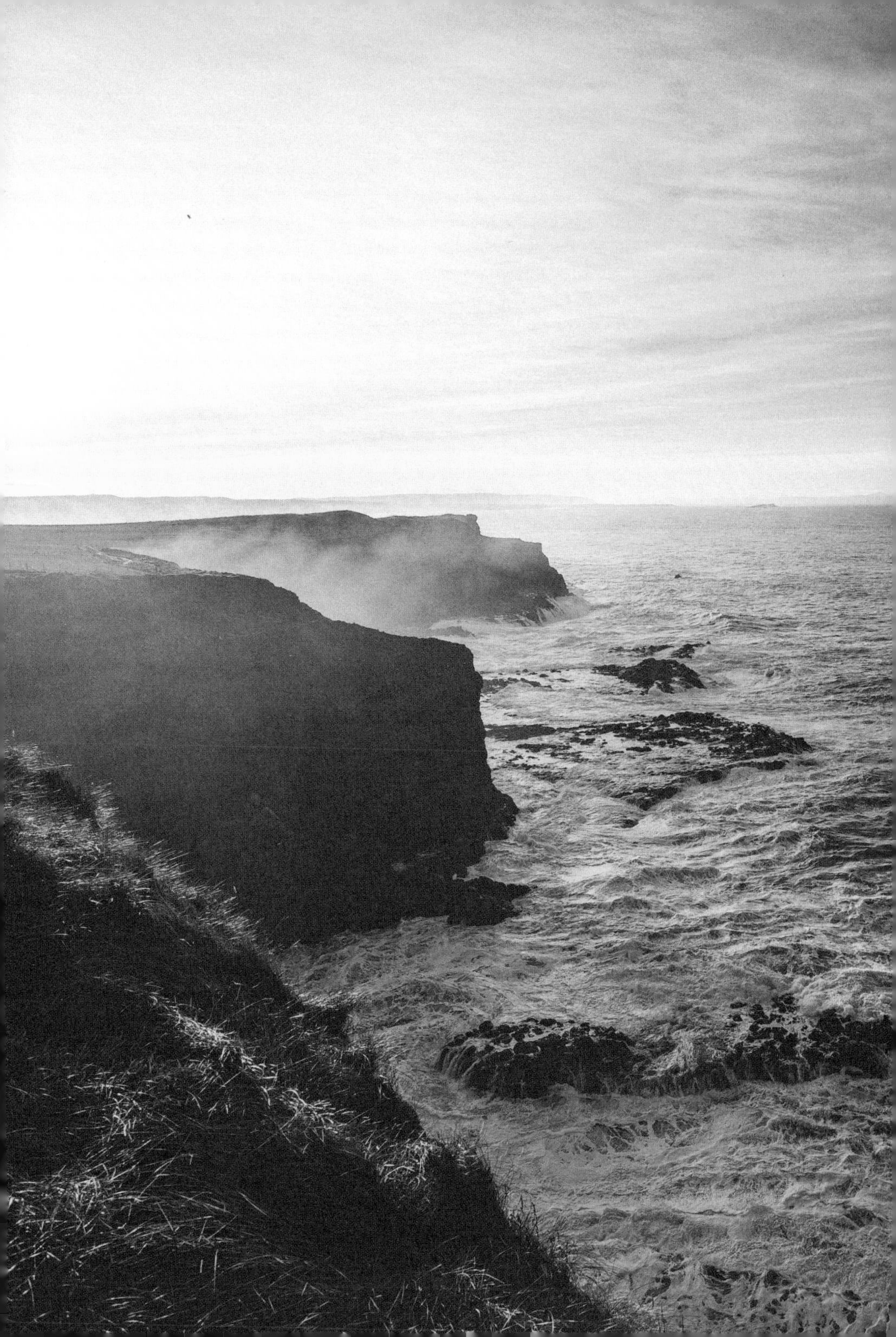

PRACTISING MINDFULNESS

Whatever else you plan to do at the beach, try to spend some of your time simply being. Mindfulness, the act of keeping your mind and attention in the present – on the sights, sounds and smells around you – helps prevent thoughts ruminating and gives your mind a break. Scientific research in this area is growing rapidly because those who practise mindfulness report that it helps reduce stress and anxiety and improves mood.

Aim to immerse yourself in the coastal environment and really appreciate where you are. Turn off your phone so you can bathe your senses in the stimulation around you without fear of distraction. If your mind starts to wander – pondering problems at work, what you are going to make for dinner, whether you left the iron on – keep bringing it back to the here and now and see if you can stay present without getting lost in thoughts. Every time it wanders (and it will), just calmly bring it back, without judgement.

Take off your shoes and walk on the beach barefoot, even if it's a little chilly. It can be a powerful sensation to physically connect with your surroundings. It really will make you feel grounded. Aim to use all five senses (see pages 95–7) to explore the environment around you, really noticing the small details.

Listen

- Close your eyes and listen to the sound of the sea. The slow, churning, white noise of the ocean can be comforting. Is the sound loud or quiet? Does the sea sound calm or choppy?
- Hear the waves breaking and dispersing on the beach. Listen to the different sound the waves make as they retreat again, drawing sand or pebbles back down the beach with them. Is the frequency of the waves regular or irregular? Listen for a while to see whether you can hear if any waves are bigger than others.
- Can you hear the cries of gulls or any other sea birds? Are they all the same type or are there different calls? Can you hear any other living creatures?
- It is often breezy at the coast, sometimes positively windy. Listen to the sound of the wind swishing around your face and body and making a rustling sound through your hair. Is the wind blowing consistently or in gusts?
- What other sounds can you hear? Take a few moments to identify the individual noises. Can you hear people talking or dogs barking? What is the furthest sound you can hear?

Taste

- Stand facing the breeze with your eyes closed. Open your mouth and taste the air. Can you taste salt on your tongue? Your tongue should capture the salt from the sea spray circulating in the air.
- Now lick your lips. Do they taste salty too? If you've been exercising on the beach or have had an energetic walk, can you notice a slight bitter taste of sweat on your top lip?
- If you've brought a picnic to the beach, eat slowly with your eyes closed to really taste what you're eating. Don't just wolf the food down automatically. Try to identify individual flavours in the foods you are eating.
- If you can get organized, bring a selection of snacks with you to taste at the beach – sour gherkins or pickles, sweet berries, salty olives or chunks of cheese, bitter dark chocolate. Really concentrate as you taste them and feel their effect on your tongue.
- Slowly sip the water you've brought to the beach and notice it has never tasted crisper, cooler or fresher than it does right now.

Touch

- Stand near the sea with bare feet and feel the temperature of the sand or pebbles beneath your toes. Do they feel warm or cool? Now step nearer the sea and let a wave break over your feet. Is the water warmer or cooler? On sunny days, the water in rock pools and sandy pools will feel warmer than the sea.
- Pick up a selection of pebbles and shells from the beach. Sit down and feel the textures with your fingers and thumbs. Are the pebbles smoother than the shells? Now rub them gently on your cheeks to see whether you can feel the difference.
- If it's a sandy beach, take a handful of dry sand and let it run through your fingers, feeling the grains falling. Compare a handful of wet sand and dry sand. How different do the textures feel? Is one heavier than the other?
- Sit down and move the sand through the spaces between your toes. Feel the different textures of the smooth sand, the tiny pebbles and the pieces of shell. Is the sand soft and powdery, or rough and abrasive?
- If there are rocks on the beach, do they feel rough and craggy – even sharp – or smooth and worn down by the sea? Run your hand over them and feel the texture. If there is seaweed growing on the rocks, does it feel silky and smooth, or slimy to the touch?

See

- See the rhythmic pattern of the waves as they form out in the sea, slowly get bigger and build strength as they move towards the beach, then break on the shore. Watch for waves of different sizes – are some bigger than others?
- Watch the delicate salt spray billowing up as each wave hits the beach. Stand in the shallow water and watch the sand or small pebbles under your feet moving forward and backward as the waves come in and out.
- Look further out to sea. Can you see any boats? See the horizon where the sky kisses the sea. Can you see where the sky ends and the sea begins?
- See the different colours on the beach, the subtly different shades of the pebbles and the shells, the colour of the sand. Now look for bright colours: coastal flowers, beach towels, parasols.
- Watch as sea birds fly low over the ocean or soar up into the sky on a current of warm air. Search for movement in rock pools – can you see any living creatures?
- If it's a windy day, see the wind catching the tops of the cresting waves and creating spray. The direction of the wind can change through the course of the day (tending to be an onshore sea breeze early in the morning and an offshore land breeze later in the day). If you are at the beach all day, see if the wind shifts and how it affects the spray on the wave crests.

Smell

- When you first arrive at the beach, take a few deep breaths and smell the salty air. Sea air has a refreshing, organic aroma.
- Can you identify any other smells in the air? Close your eyes and breathe deeply and slowly. Suntan lotion, wet dog and fried food and are all common seaside smells.
- Smell your skin before and after you bathe. Does dry skin have a different smell to wet skin? Does wet hair smell different to dry hair?
- The green, herbaceous smell of seaweed will also emanate from the rock pools. The smell will be even stronger if the tide is out and the seaweed is exposed to the sun.
- If you have brought a picnic with you, enjoy the aromas of the food before and as you eat. Although they are separate senses, taste and smell are closely entwined, working together to enhance our perceptions of food.

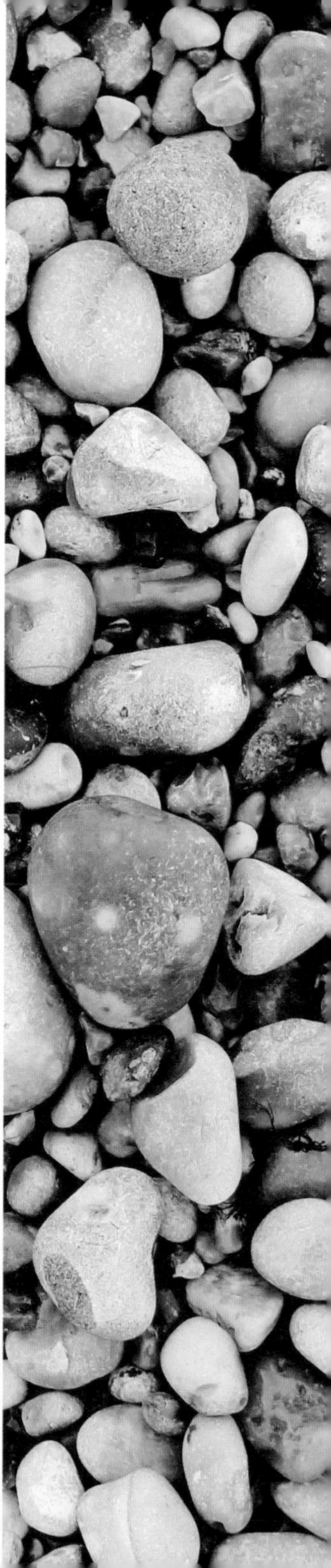

Take a Mindful Stroll

1. Slip off your shoes and start at the top of the beach. Feel the way the dry sand moves under your feet as you walk slowly along the beach. Walk on your heels for a while, pressing them into the sand, then walk on your toes and look at the difference in your footprints.

2. Now sit down in the dry sand, pick up a handful of sand and let it run through your fingers, watching the individual grains falling. Feel the temperature of the sand – is it warmer on the surface than just below?

3. If you are on a pebbly beach, pick up and feel the weight of a few of the pebbles. Can you guess which will be heavier just by looking at them? Look at the colours of the stones and the different types of rock. Can you find one with a hole right through, or some crystals embedded in it?

4. Lie down on your back with feet slightly apart and your arms a little distance from your body. Let your whole body relax. Feel the supportive quality of the beach as your body settles into it. Allow your muscles to release any tension as you let go of thoughts and simply come into the physical present. Stay in this position for as long as you like.

5. When you are ready, stand up slowly and walk down towards the sea: does the wet sand feel different and cooler under your soles? Look at your footprints in the sand as you saunter along the shore line. Can you make out each of your toes in the prints?

6. Stand for a moment and watch the waves coming in and breaking on the shore. See the way they smooth the sand. Are there small shells and pebbles embedded in the sand? Find a pebble or shell that is moving in and out with the ebb and flow of the waves. Track it to see how far it moves.

7. Look out toward the horizon and count how many shades of blue you can see on the surface of the sea. Is the sky a different blue to the sea?

8. Step into the shallow water. Does it feel warm or cool on your skin? Stand still and feel the movement of the waves against your legs. Can you feel sand being washed away under the soles of your feet as the waves go out?

9. Bend down and wet your hand. Does the back of your wet hand smell different to your dry hand? Lick your hand and taste the tang of salt.

BEACH ACTIVITIES

It's tempting to sit back in a comfy beach chair and immerse yourself in a good book, but it's far more beneficial to look around you and be inspired by your surroundings. The idea is to bathe in the atmosphere of the coastal environment and reap the rewards. Here are a few activities to help you really focus on what's around you.

Rock-pooling

Rock-pooling is a popular family activity at the beach. It is an excellent way for both children and adults to experience and connect with nature, and to gain an appreciation of how fascinating nature can be.

If the beach you visit has rock pools, get in there and explore them. You will be surprised at just how many fascinating creatures you can find in such a small space, and all the beautiful seaweeds there. Take a small net and a bucket if you want to examine them up close, but be sure to return them to the pool in which you found them. See page 178 for some guidelines on responsible rock-pooling.

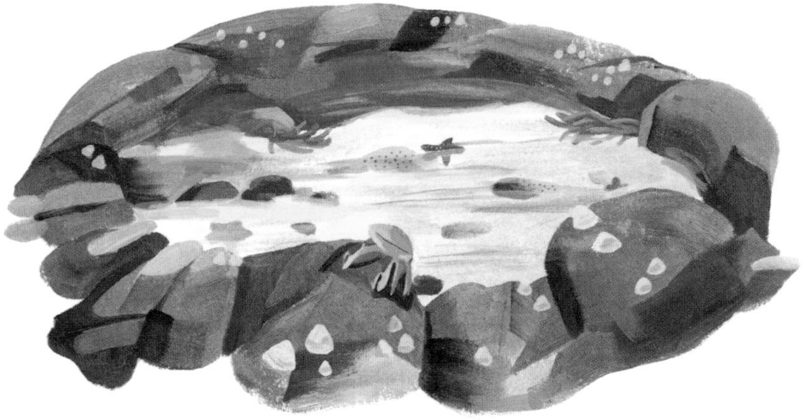

Fun in the Sand

Sandcastles aren't just for kids. Try your hand at a sand sculpture, making it as simple or adventurous as you like. Use your imagination – small pebbles, shells, driftwood and seaweed can add decoration or features.

Get Creative

Being in a natural environment really does boost creativity so look around and get inspired. Painting, drawing and creative writing are all great activities for the beach, allowing you to connect even more deeply with your surroundings. Nobody else needs to see your work if you feel self-conscious about it – just enjoy the process and its restorative benefits.

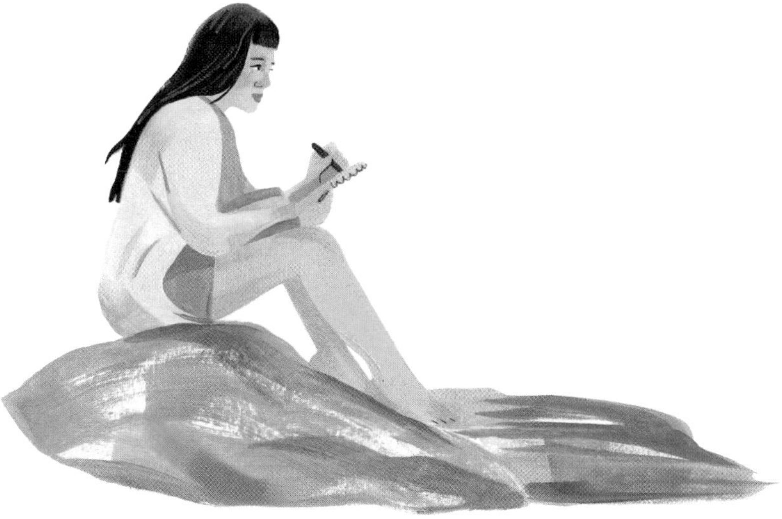

Wildlife Watching

All beaches are suitable for watching wildlife, but the type will depend on where you are. Take guide books and binoculars or simply have a look around you to see what you can see – birds, crabs, sea mammals. A nature walk along the beach offers a good opportunity for exercise and can allow you to appreciate a range of different habits, such as the shoreline, sand dunes, marshes or estuary. See pages 176–7 for some guidelines on responsible wildlife watching.

Collecting Sea Glass

Collecting sea glass (small pieces of broken glass which have been smoothed by the action of the sea) offers a good excuse for taking a stroll, improving fitness levels. Walking on sand uses up more calories than walking on a firm surface, and walking on sand with bare feet works a whole range of different muscles. As a bonus, the sand will smooth the skin on your feet as you walk.

Meditating

Use the sound of the waves or your breathing to help you meditate (see pages 106–7). The outdoor natural setting will enhance the relaxation effects. Or try some breathing exercises to relax you (see pages 108–9).

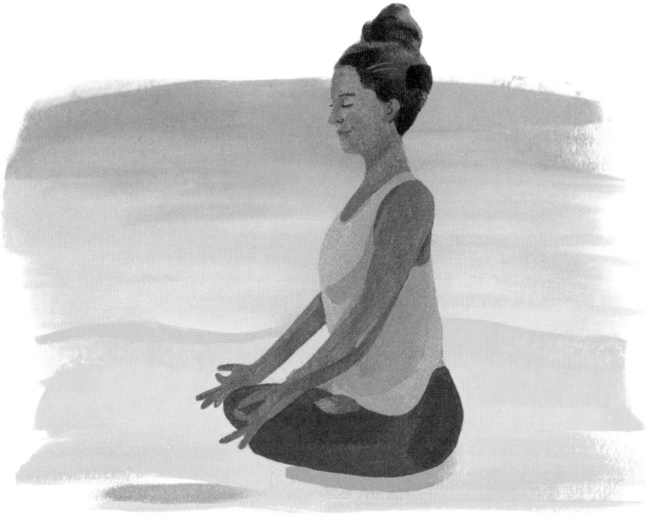

Picnics

A picnic is a great reason to visit the beach, and taking food with you will increase the time you can spend there. Friends and family can turn the trip into a relaxing social occasion. A picnic breakfast at sunrise or drinks at sunset will inspire feelings of awe.

Working Out

A natural setting makes exercise more enjoyable, and may even make it feel a little easier (see pages 111–15). The sand and water offer extra challenges, and can reduce stress on the joints. Whether you want a gentle stroll or a full-body workout, the beach is a good location.

Contact with Water

Any physical connection with the sea – paddling, swimming, diving under the waves, surfing or body boarding – will increase your psychological connection to the natural environment. These activities also offer physical benefits in terms of exercise and possible benefits in terms of immersion in magnesium-rich salt water (see pages 43 and 129).

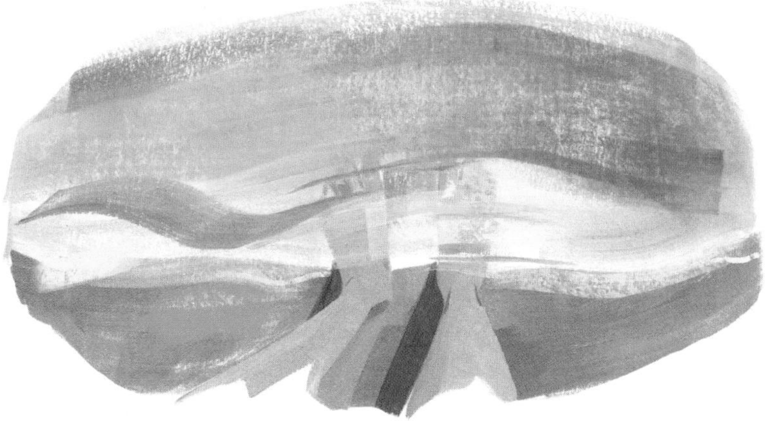

Floating

Studies into the benefits of flotation therapy (see page 136) have shown that floating in salt water lowers levels of stress hormones, reduces blood pressure, improves sleep, helps muscles recover from exercise and aids creativity. These effects are possibly due to the magnesium in the water and the sensory deprivation involved. We can assume that floating in sea water would offer some of the same benefits, so a session simply floating on your back in the sea could be beneficial. But be aware of tides and currents, to make sure you don't drift out to sea.

Stargazing

Not many of us visit the beach at night, yet this can be a hugely awe-inspiring experience. Choose a clear night and lay on your back on a towel on the sand. Make sure you are comfortable, folding another towel to act as a pillow or covering yourself with a blanket if it's chilly. Listen to the waves breaking on the shore as you gaze up at the stars above. Be sure to check the tide times before you go.

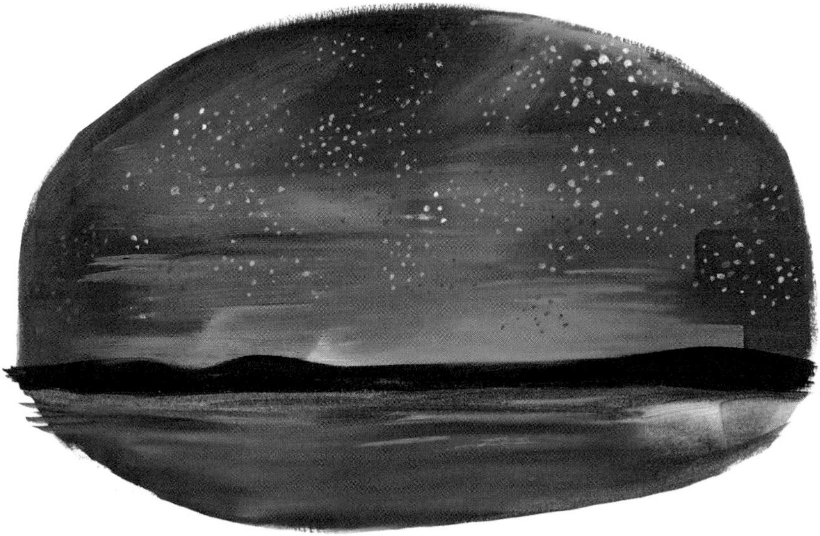

Enjoying Seafood

Collecting and eating some of the edible species around you – shellfish, shrimps, seaweed, coastal plants such as samphire – will increase your psychological connection to nature and offer health benefits too. These are some of the most nutritious foods on the planet. It is sensible to refer to a seashore foraging handbook, or take part in an organized foraging course, to advise you what to collect and where, and to avoid possible contamination. These sources may also introduce you to some new recipes for your finds. Be sure to check local regulations and limits on the collection of seafood or, alternatively, find a restaurant offering local catches.

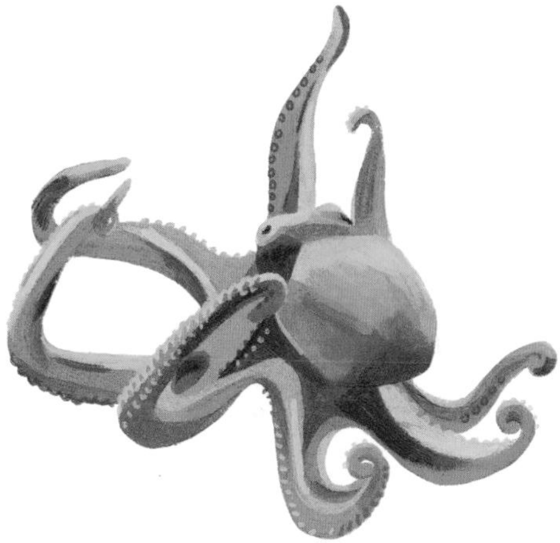

MEDITATION BY THE SEA

Regular meditation can help reduce stress, build self-confidence and self-esteem, and maintain good health. Meditating on the beach is even better, as it allows you to connect with nature while also providing the perfect soundtrack to focus on – the sound of the waves. Perhaps one of the greatest benefits of meditation is that it can give your mind a break from overthinking and rumination, something we all do from time to time.

For many people, regular meditation doesn't sound that appealing, just another thing you don't have time to do, and it's not always easy to begin. Yet when you meditate, your body undergoes physiological changes that result in lower blood pressure, an improved immune system, a decrease in tension-related pain (like headaches or muscle pain), increased energy and increased production of serotonin (the happy hormone).

If the physical reasons aren't enough, there are some amazing psychological benefits to meditating as well, including decreased anxiety and tension, increased creativity and happiness, and a sharpening of the mind and ability to focus. Here are two easy meditations to try.

Sound of the Waves Meditation

This mindfulness practice uses the sound of the waves on the beach as an object to focus the attention on.

1. Sit comfortably near the water's edge in an alert upright position. Close your eyes and relax your body, including your face and shoulders. Let all the tension go, while still maintaining your posture and alignment.

2. Once you are settled, turn your awareness to your breath. Breathe deeply in and out for a minute or two, noticing the sound and frequency of your breath but not trying to change it.

3. Now gently bring your attention to the sound of the waves. Notice each wave as it breaks on the shore, then retreats – in and out, in and out. Really focus.

4. When you notice your mind starts to wander, as it most certainly will, gently bring your attention back to the sound of the waves. Continue for 10 minutes.

Water Visualization Meditation

This meditation uses visualization to focus the mind. Use the sound of the waves to help really conjure the image of water in your mind.

1. Sit comfortably near the water's edge in an alert upright position. Close your eyes and relax your body, including your face and shoulders. Let all the tension go, while still maintaining your posture and alignment.

2. Once you are settled, turn your awareness to your breath. Think of your breath as water; it can flow freely, filling whatever space it enters. Breathe in softly, visualizing the air entering your body like a wave that is flowing onto the shore. The wave – your breath – continues to flow as long as it can remain whole without faltering.

3. At the top of your breath, pause for a moment, just as the wave does before the water starts to soak into the sand.

4. When you begin to release your breath, let it go gently like ocean water soaking into the sand. The water disappears smoothly and evenly. Allow your exhalation to spread through your body the same way. Your body will relax like sand on the shore changing from dry to wet.

5. At the end of the exhalation, pause briefly before the next wave or breath begins. Continue for 10 minutes, gently bringing your attention back to the visualization if your mind wanders.

RELAXING BREATHING EXERCISES

Breathing is key to sustaining life yet we are rarely conscious of it. Research shows that conscious breathing can help reduce stress, regulate emotions, improve sleep and reduce cravings. Try these simple breathing exercises to calm your mind and help you think clearly. They can be done anywhere, but a natural setting – such as a beach – will enhance their benefits.

Simple Breath Awareness

Simple breath awareness is a gentle diaphragmatic breathing technique which, as the name suggests, makes you more aware of your breath. It can help to calm the nervous system, reduce stress and enhance awareness.

1. Lay on your back on your towel, sit on a beach chair or sit cross-legged on the sand. Close your eyes and lay your hands lightly on your stomach.
2. Breathe at a normal rate in and out of your nose for 1 minute, observing the quality of the breath.
3. Try not to judge how you are breathing – simply observe it.
4. If you find your breath is tense or shallow, relax all parts of your body, including your face and tongue, and pause at the beginning and the end of each breath.
5. Continue for another 2–4 minutes, observing each breath.

Alternate Nostril Breathing

This is a yoga breathing technique which takes a little practice to master but offers a great opportunity for mindfulness and relaxation.

1. Sit comfortably on the sand or on a beach chair and place your left hand, palm facing down, on your left knee. Place your right hand on your right leg, palm facing up, and tuck your index and middle fingers into your palm, leaving the other fingers extended.
2. Inhale and exhale deeply for a count of 10, then place your right thumb over your right nostril. Inhale again slowly through your left nostril.
3. Hold your breath for a count of 3 then place your ring finger over your left nostril. Release your thumb, then slowly exhale out through your right nostril.

4. Inhale through your right nostril, then place your thumb over your right nostril and hold your breath for a count of 3.
5. Release your ring finger then exhale out through your left nostril. You have completed one full cycle.
6. Repeat 5–10 cycles with your eyes closed, then return your right hand to your right knee and sit at ease for a moment, enjoying the feeling of calm.

Ocean Breathing

If you do it correctly, this breathing technique sounds like waves on the ocean. If your mind has a habit of wandering, this exercise will help bring your attention back to the moment. Just focus on how your breath feels and sounds.

1. Stand in a comfortable position or sit cross-legged on the sand. Take a few deep inhalations and exhalations through your nose and relax your whole body.
2. Bring one of your hands up in front of your face with your palm facing you, and exhale onto your palm through your mouth as if you were trying to fog up a mirror.
3. Inhale, then keeping your hand in front of your face, exhale in the same way again but this time with your mouth closed so the air comes out through your nose. You will feel a slight constricting sensation in the back of your throat and hear a sound like an ocean wave.
4. Bring your hand down to your side, close your eyes and continue breathing in through the nose normally, and out through the nose with the rushing sound, for 5 minutes.

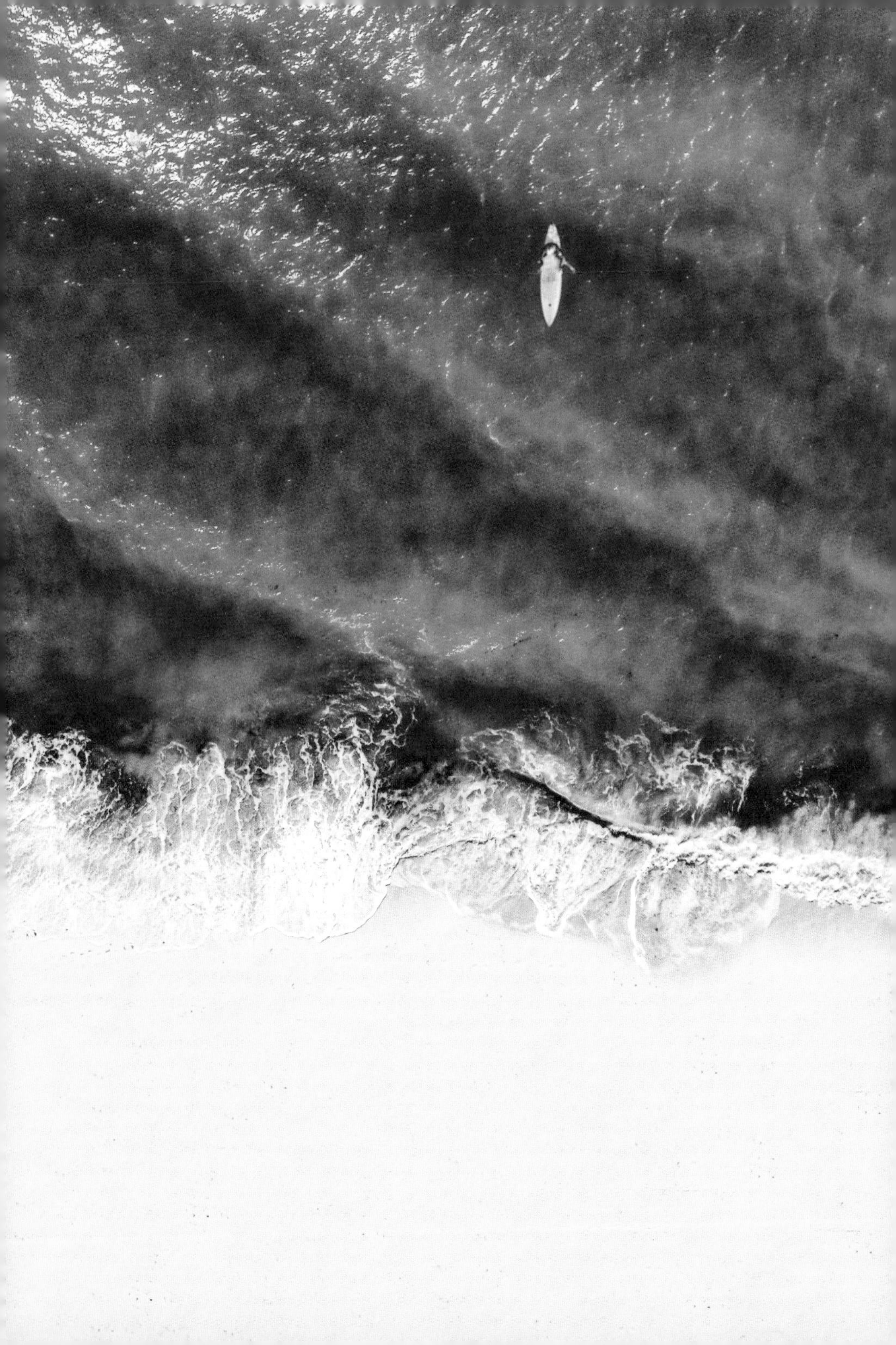

EXERCISING AT THE BEACH

Many studies have shown that exercising in a natural environment offers greater benefits, both physical and psychological, than exercising indoors (see pages 46–54). The term "green exercise" was first coined in 2003 to describe a physical activity performed while simultaneously being exposed to nature. Most studies have been conducted in countryside or woodland, but it seems the effect is the same whatever the natural environment, beaches included.[144] One study even suggested that the presence of water generated greater effects.[76]

IN THE WATER

Exercising in water offers the easiest form of aerobic activity for elderly people, individuals with joint pain or arthritis, or those who have recently undergone surgery. The water effectively reduces the weight of a person by 90 per cent, allowing them to exercise without impact, taking the stress off the joints.

Exercising in water builds cardiovascular stamina, strength and flexibility. It helps burn body fat, increases circulation and can help rehabilitate healing muscles and joints. You might think you can't get as intense a workout in water, but research suggests otherwise. Due to the resistance of the water, it just seems like you can't work as hard, but in reality you are. And because water lessens the effects of gravity, you're able to move your body through a wider range of motion, which improves flexibility. Even your lungs get a beneficial workout, because the water pressure makes them work harder than they would on land.

Because it's low impact and easily tailored to your fitness level, anyone can benefit from exercising in water. It's the ideal choice on a warm day as the water will cool you down as you work.

Swimming

Swimming is a great way to exercise, whatever your age or level of fitness. Recreational swimming burns about the same number of calories as brisk walking but because the water supports your weight, it's much less stressful on the joints. It can be the ideal exercise for people who are overweight, or those with knee or ankle problems. The water offers resistance as you move through it so you can work as hard as you like with little chance of injury.

The act of swimming can be relaxing and meditative, so it offers stress relief as well as cardiovascular benefits. If you haven't been swimming for a while, start with just 5–10 minutes, concentrating on coordinating your breathing with your strokes. A pair of goggles will protect your eyes from the seawater, and be sure to check for currents and undertow before you begin. Whether you choose to don flippers and a snorkel to explore the sea life, or just swim around the bay, swimming is great exercise.

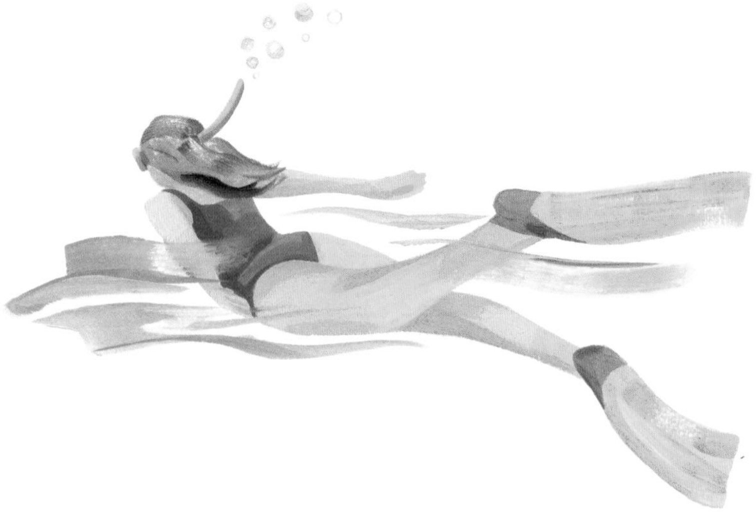

Aqua Jogging

Aqua jogging is similar to running on land, but without the joint impact. It can be done in deep water with a flotation device to support your body, or in shoulder-depth water where you can reach the bottom. Simply run on the spot, bringing your knees up high and leaning slightly forward. Continue until you have set a regular rhythm, going fast enough to raise your heart rate. Maintain the rhythm for as long as you can.

For extra benefit, you can include your arms in the exercise. Lift your left arm up as you lift your right knee, keeping your shoulders still and bending your elbow to about a 90-degree angle. Extend the arm back down as the knee goes down, then lift your right arm at the same time as your left knee. This exercise works the biceps, triceps and lower abdominals.

Surfing and Body Boarding

These more strenuous activities offer total immersion – both literally and metaphorically – in the environment of the sea, allowing all five senses to experience it to the full. They can create a real sense of "getting away from it all" into another world (see page 33), both when coping with the waves and currents and physical immersion in the sea itself, and when looking back towards land from a position of relative isolation out to sea. This may enable more objective reflection on life's problems and engender a sense of calm.

Although the physicality of these sports might seem offputting to some, being pummelled by the waves can offer emotional benefits as well as physical ones. In a study of combat veterans experiencing post-traumatic stress disorder, some of the participants reported that they felt the pummelling of the waves "washed away" their negative emotions. Surfing enabled the veterans to push PTSD into the background and experience a sense of respite from symptoms. It also helped to prevent them feeling overwhelmed by their suffering.[145]

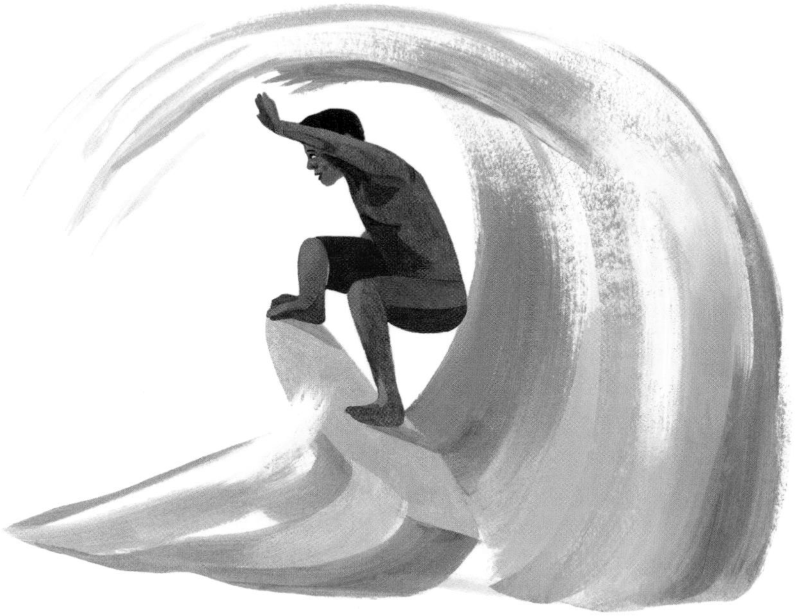

ON THE SAND

Exercising on sand is harder than exercising on a solid surface. The sand gives as you push off so you use more strength and energy in any activity you do. It results in a more demanding workout, burning more calories and building more muscle. The sand also absorbs some of your weight as you land, which reduces the stress on your joints, particularly your knees, hips and ankles.

The beach is the ideal place for a wide range of activities, including skipping, frisbee, beach volleyball, running or a full workout. Or simply take a stroll along the water's edge – any kind of exercise will be enhanced by the action of the sand. Unless you are very fit, position yourself close to the water where the sand is more stable. Move up the beach on to softer sand if you want more of a challenge. Any exercise you do will be made more difficult because of the uneven and sinking surface.

When exercising on the beach, don't let the cool sea breeze fool you into thinking it's cooler than it is. Don't underestimate the impact of the temperature and UV radiation on your body and avoid exercising in the midday sun. Mornings and evenings are the best time to exercise on the beach. Make sure you drink plenty of water throughout the day, wear a hat and apply sunscreen in the middle of the day.

Simple Stretches

Stretching feels good and offers a range of benefits, both physical and mental. Most animals stretch frequently throughout the day, yet it's not something we as humans do very often. A few simple stretches will help release tension, clearing your mind and making you feel more in touch with your body. Regular stretching can increase coordination, flexibility and improve the range of motion in your joints, helping you move more freely.

For maximum benefit, warm up with 5–10 minutes of light activity before stretching, perhaps taking a stroll down the beach. Or better still, try a few stretches after a workout. Aim to work on as many of your muscles as possible. Keep the stretches gentle and slow; only stretch as deep as is comfortable. Don't jerk or bounce. Breathe steadily through your stretches and if you feel any pain, you've stretched too far. The stretch should feel good and shouldn't hurt.

Walking and Running

Compared to walking or running on a pavement or grass, walking or running on sand is much harder, but also more effective. The sand gives way when you push off, so some of the energy that is usually transferred to the next step is lost. This means the muscles in your feet and legs have to work much harder. You also have to engage the stabilizing muscles of your abdomen to compensate for the uneven surface so you develop a natural and very efficient walking or running style while working your core muscles. It's not surprising that many top runners train on sand.

After a more vigorous workout, your muscles will use more energy after your walk or run in order to recover properly. So they burn more calories than usual, which is known as the after-burn effect. Don't underestimate how much harder the sand makes the exercise – take it slowly and be sure to do a few stretches to warm up the muscles in your soles, calves and hamstrings before you begin.

It's tempting to walk or run barefoot on the beach, but be careful: the muscles in your feet are probably not used to this much effort so it's a good idea to start in your shoes and take them off for the last 10 or 15 minutes if you like. Stick to the wet, more compacted sand near the water's edge so your feet don't sink in as far, and keep an eye out for sharp pebbles, shells or driftwood.

CHAPTER 5

Bringing the Ocean Closer to Home

"I could never stay long enough on the shore; the tang of the untainted, fresh, and free sea air was like a cool, quieting thought."

— Helen Keller

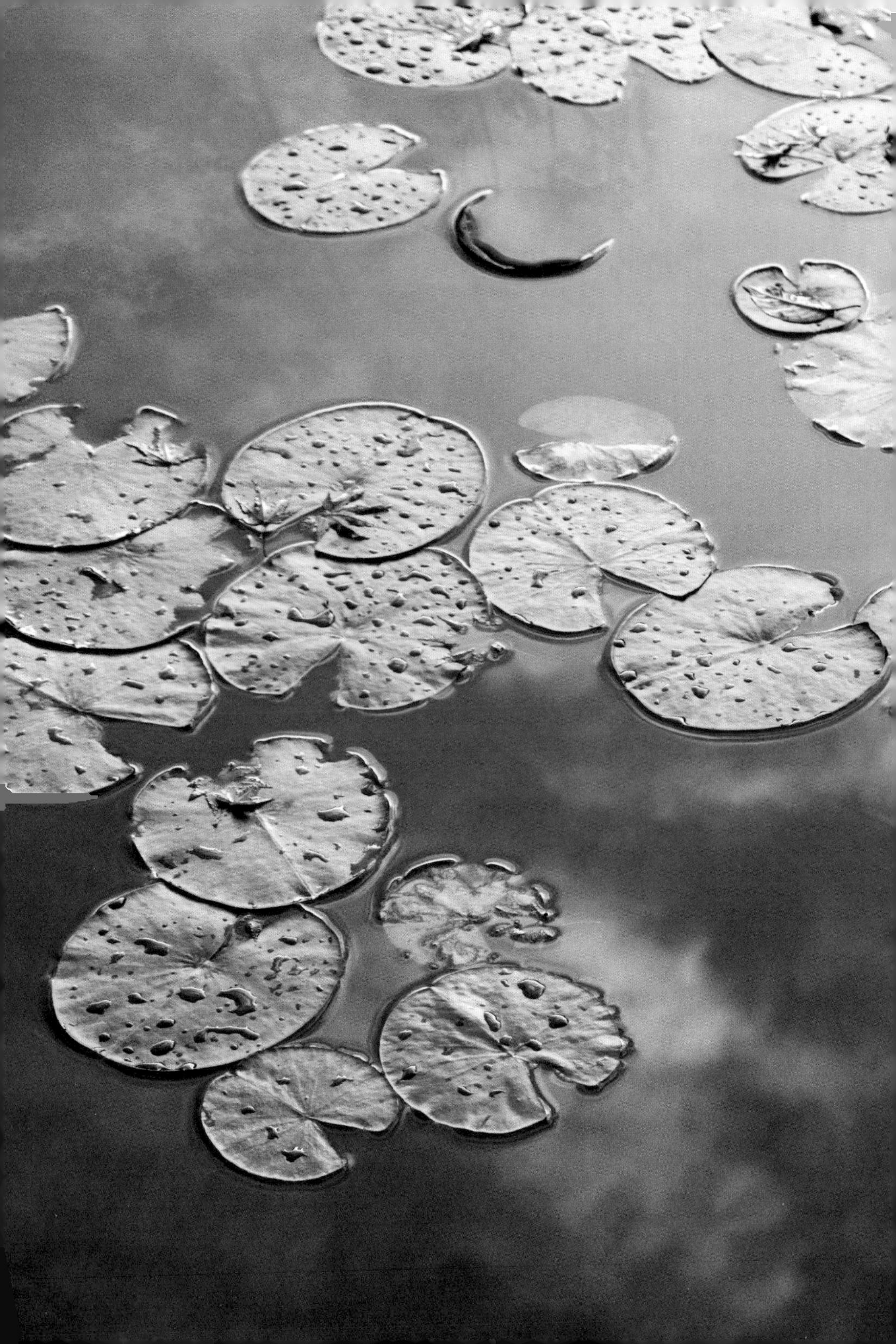

A day spent at the coast can offer a wide range of physiological and psychological benefits, but we can't always be there as often as we'd like. For many of us, daily commitments can prevent us enjoying regular leisure time, and there will be situations when access to the sea is simply not possible – for the elderly or hospitalized, for instance, and for those who are simply located too far from the coast for regular access to be practical, there may be no possibility of breathing in the fresh sea air, listening to the sea birds or staring at the ocean.

However, keeping fish at home (see page 82) or visiting public aquariums (see pages 76–7) have been found to improve mood and decrease stress – even a computer screensaver of a virtual aquarium or tropical beach can provide a measure of relaxation while at the office. And there are other ways to reap some of the beneficial effects of the ocean closer to home – whether it's a picnic by a lake, a salt water bath, a seaweed face mask or a wonderful plate of highly nutritious grilled sardines.

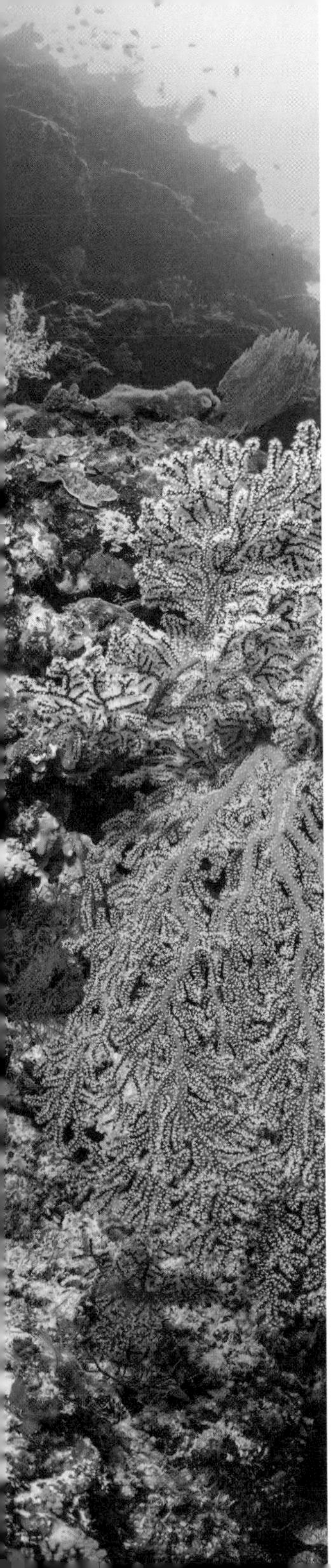

USING VIRTUAL REALITY

Studies now suggest that exposure to a virtual environment may provide at least some of the benefits of being by the sea.[3, 115] Virtual reality (VR) is a term that describes a three-dimensional, computer-generated environment that a person can explore and interact with.[146] While often associated with recreational uses and career training (for example flight simulators), VR has also been used for the psychological and medical treatment of many human conditions, such as helping people overcome phobias or as a distraction therapy for the control of pain.[147]

Virtual Restorative Environments

VR is becoming increasingly available in healthcare settings and researchers are beginning to work with clinicians to explore the use of Virtual Restorative Environments (VREs) – scenes of natural beauty or peacefulness that can help to reduce stress and anxiety, or assist recovery from mental fatigue.[147] One study, for instance, used a marine VRE – consisting of a coastal path with views of the sea, a beach and nearby fields – to explore how interacting with virtual nature could influence and alleviate the experience of dental pain.

The researchers found that the dental patients who experienced the virtual coast path reported feeling less pain compared with those patients viewing urban VR, or just receiving the standard dental care.[148] Marine VREs have also been used to help patients in physical rehabilitation programmes. Using a virtual marine environment, combined with interactive features, can aid recovery from surgical procedures and specifically help amputees to undertake competitive and motivational virtual exercises. These interactive and dynamic exercises can help amputees avoid muscle atrophy while they are waiting for their prosthetic limbs to be fitted.[147]

Real Blue Environments

Other types of virtual environment are also being researched. For instance, the BlueHealth project[149] (see page 89) is using 360-degree cameras to take footage of real blue environments with the aim of letting people who cannot access a "real environment" experience the environment virtually. High-quality 360-degree video footage of a variety of blue environments will be taken from land, air and underwater, and will contain a suite of different scenes – from calming beaches to vibrant and stimulating coral reefs – which will provide a range of possible experiences. It is hoped that these pre-recorded videos may be able to improve the wellbeing of those unable to access the real environment, perhaps because they are elderly and are confined to a care home, or because they have physical impairments which prevent them from being able to access the real environment. That way everyone should be able to experience the benefits of being by the sea, either in reality or virtually.

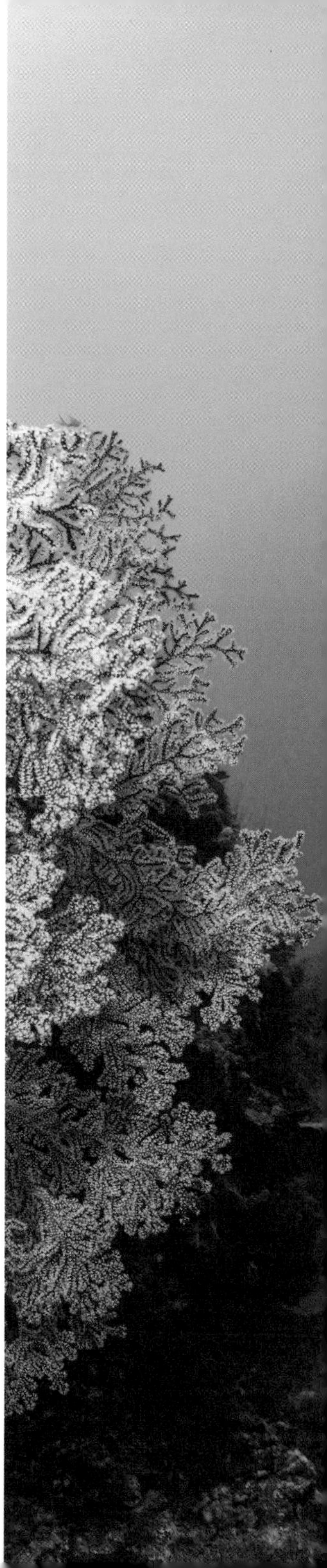

Water in Urban Settings

While few experiences can beat the relaxing and stress-busting effects of a day at the coast – when we literally "get away from it all" – water in the urban landscape could offer something in the way of a substitution. As cities grow larger and swallow up open spaces, most of us have fewer opportunities to engage with nature and enjoy its restorative qualities. Urban planners are beginning to recognize the benefits to health and wellbeing of incorporating natural features into the built environment – parks, gardens, pockets of wasteland, and particularly water features.

Water has played a huge part in the design of gardens and public spaces throughout history, from the Hanging Gardens of Babylon through to modern times, and has long been appreciated for its aesthetic properties. Humans are drawn to water and fascinated by it: we picnic by lakes, ponds and fountains, or simply sit and gaze at them when we get the chance. They can offer the ideal place for meeting and relaxing in an urban environment. Look at any city and you'll find people gathered around fountains in squares, or strolling along a waterfront.

Many studies have demonstrated how highly we prize water – such as lakes, ponds and rivers – in a landscape and how it makes us feel. One study[150] showed that when they were asked whether they liked photographs of landscapes (both urban and natural), people rated the landscapes containing water much more highly than those without water (see pages 28–9). In fact, they rated scenes of urban landscapes that contained water as highly as the natural landscapes without water and reported that the landscapes with water made them feel better and were perceived as more restorative than those without.

Other studies have shown that the degree of "naturalness" affects how much we like a scene containing water. The larger the area of water, the more we tend to like it, and we are especially drawn to water with natural vegetation growing around the edges or areas of water surrounded by boulders or rocks, and with an informal curved shape. All these characteristics lead to a greater feeling of tranquillity within us. So if you don't have the opportunity to escape to the coast, seek out a lake, pond or river near to where you live and plan a walk or picnic there.

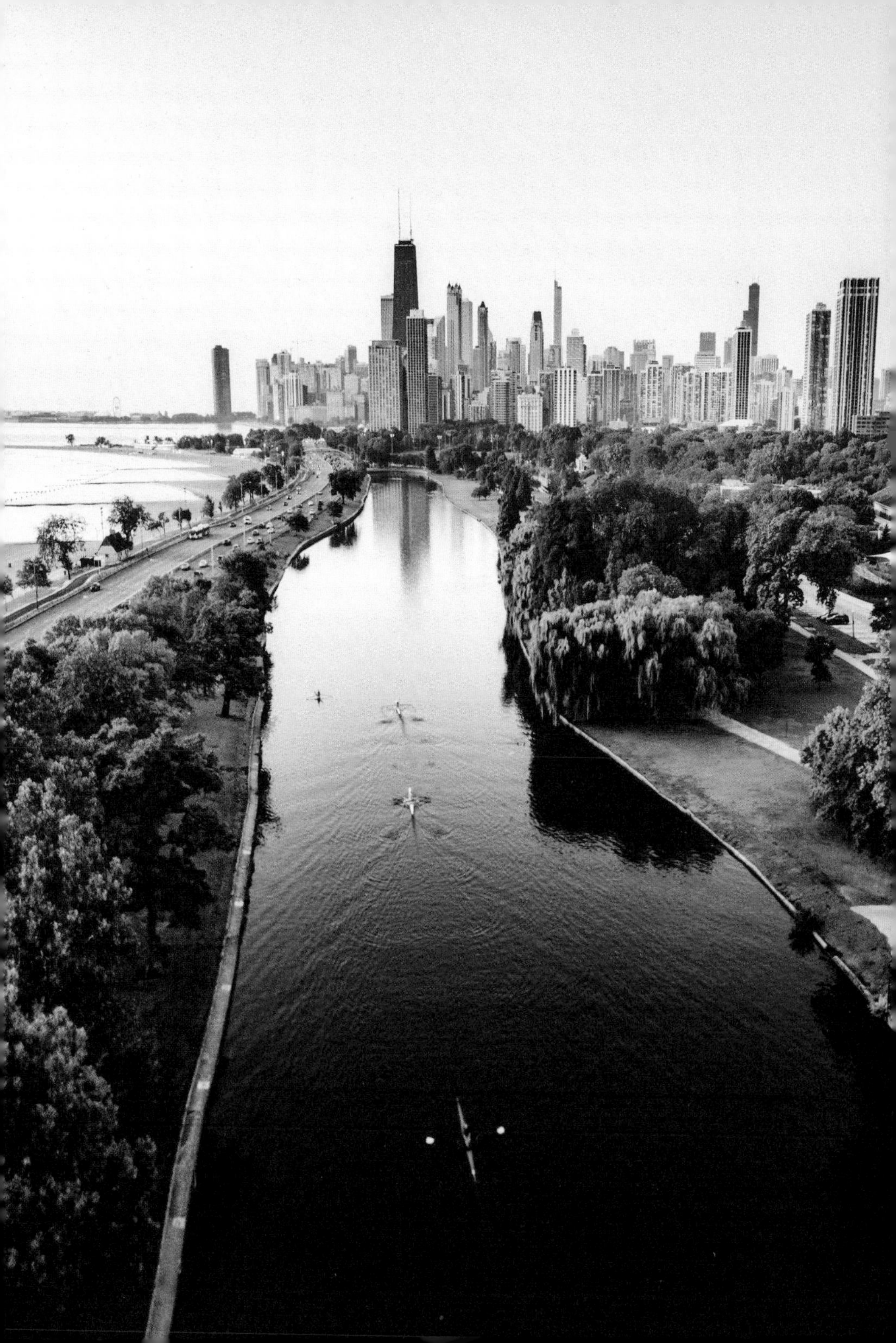

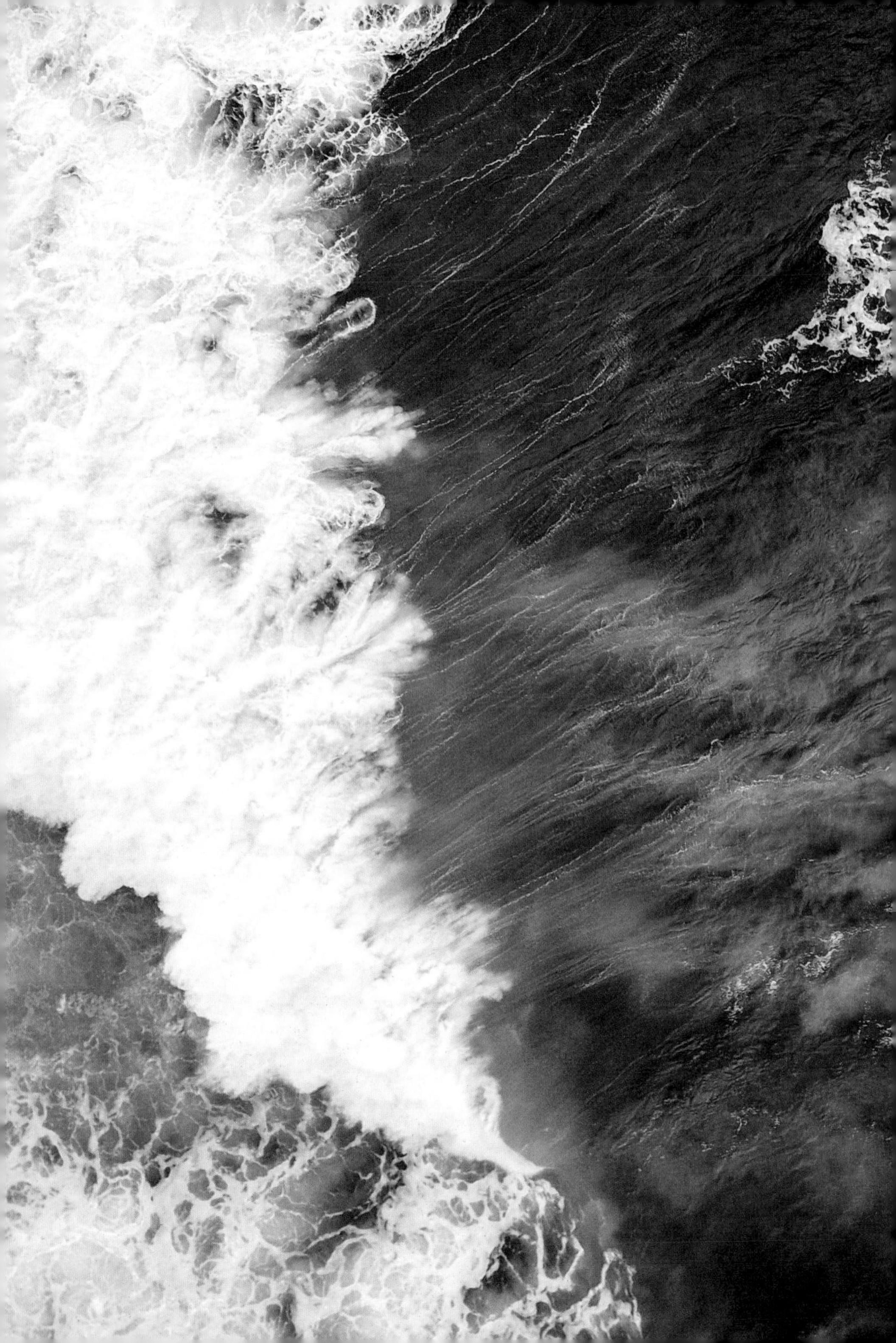

Relaxing Wave Sounds

Research shows that the sound of ocean waves alters the wave patterns in our brains, lulling us into a more relaxed state. Researchers in the UK found that listening to natural sounds affected the fight-or-flight and rest-digest autonomic nervous systems, and also affected the resting activity of the brain. When listening to natural sounds, the brain connectivity reflected an outward-directed focus of attention; when listening to artificial sounds, the brain connectivity reflected an inward-directed focus of attention, similar to states observed in anxiety, post-traumatic stress disorder and depression. There was also an increase in rest-digest nervous system activity (associated with relaxation) when listening to natural compared with artificial sounds, and participants performed better on tasks requiring concentration.[151]

WHEN TO USE WAVE SOUNDS

Soundtracks of ocean waves offer great relaxation benefits. Ocean sounds are perfect for calming activities such as reading, meditation or yoga and can help soothe periods of stress and anxiety. They are also ideal for use in the workplace, helping to improve concentration and boost creativity.

WAVE SOUNDS FOR SLEEPING

Many people find the sound of waves can help them sleep. More abrupt, artificial sounds, such as a phone ringing or traffic passing outside, are perceived by the brain as a potential threat and therefore demand attention. Slow-building sounds, like ocean waves, can be louder but don't distract the brain so they can be used to block out artificial sounds and aid sleep.

WHO CAN BENEFIT?

Wave sounds can benefit just about anyone, either to improve sleep or as an aid to relaxation, creating a calm environment and boosting wellbeing. They are helpful for soothing babies, masking outside noises and helping them sleep. Older children can use wave sounds to drown out distractions from outside noises, leading to better concentration when studying.

Ocean Visualization

This visualization can be enjoyed just about anywhere. It will help you recreate in your mind a day by the sea and, hopefully, reap some of the relaxation benefits of actually being there.

Most of us are familiar with meditation, but fewer of us with visualization. Yet it can be a powerful tool to aid relaxation, improve sleep and engender a sense of wellbeing. The idea with meditation is to give the body and mind a deep rest – doing less will help you achieve more. Visualization is more active: you guide your thoughts to visualize a scenario and use your imagination to have a five-sensory experience.

1. Gather together any items you may have that remind you of the sea – seashells, beach pebbles, sea glass, a small pot of beach sand collected on a previous visit – and spend a few minutes examining them. A recording of ocean sounds can also be a great help, but don't worry if you don't have any of these things. Just sit quietly in a comfortable position and close your eyes.

2. Take a few long, slow breaths. Let all other thoughts float away as you concentrate on your breathing. Feel the cool air coming in and the warm air going out. Don't try to change your breathing – just notice it.

3. Now mentally check your body to feel if any of your muscles are tense, paying particular attention to your face and tongue. Let all the tension melt away as you breathe in and out. Feel yourself becoming more and more comfortable and relaxed.

4. Visualize the ocean itself in your mind's eye. Allow all of your senses to participate in your mental journey:

– Feel the cool spray of sea mist on your face.
– Hear the sea's rhythmic roar as the waves come and go.
– Smell the briny tang of the ocean in the air.
– Watch the sun playing over the ocean's surface, creating shifting patches of vivid blues and greens. See the swell of the waves.
– Taste the salt on your lips.

5. Spend a few minutes drinking in the beauty of the vast ocean, stretching as far as the horizon, and allow feelings of awe to wash over you.

6. Once you are fully engaged with the setting, visualize yourself standing on the beach facing the ocean. Feel the tiny grains of soft sand under your toes and the breeze on your face. As the sun warms your back, a soothing sensation of relaxation melts through your whole body. Watch the waves as they form, break on the shore, then retreat. Hear the hypnotic sound as they break and retreat...break and retreat. The rhythmic sound calms your mind.

7. Imagine yourself stepping forward, the sand yielding a little beneath your feet and getting cooler as you approach the water. You hear the distant cries of a seagull overhead. A wave breaks over your feet. Feel the cool and refreshing water envelope your toes and ankles, the tickle of sand moving beneath your soles. Remain there feeling the waves gently and rhythmically breaking over your feet for as long as you like.

8. When you are ready, bring your attention back to your breathing and become aware of your body once again.

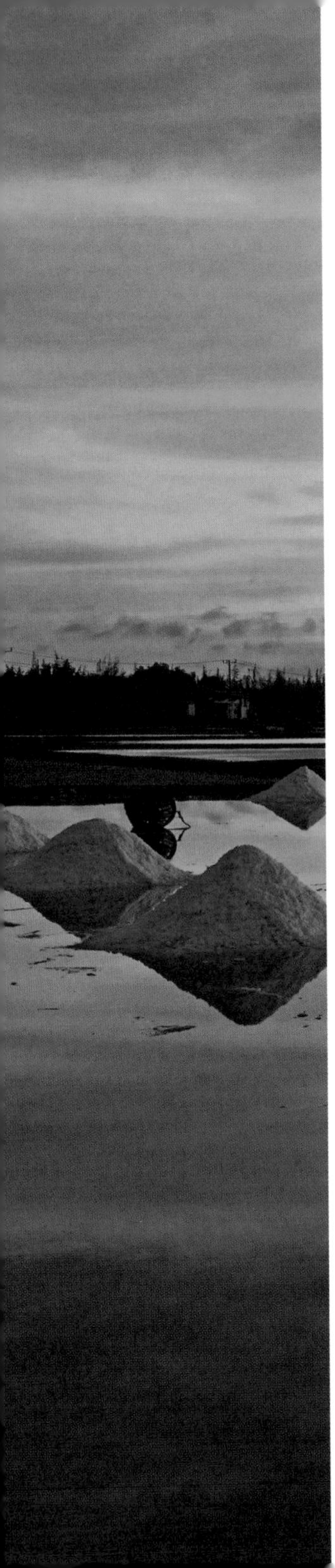

Salt Therapies at Home

Throughout history, salt has been an important source of wealth, one of the most coveted products in the world. But not just for its use in the preparation of food – salt has long been celebrated for its healing properties as well. The history of salt in healing takes us as far back as 2,700BC in China, with the publication of the *Peng-Tzao-Kan-Mu*, the earliest known work on pharmacology. This ancient book describes more than 40 varieties of salt, with directions for their extraction and uses.

In the ancient world, warm salt water was used to treat sore muscles and arthritis, and salt was used in topical solutions to treat a range of skin conditions including psoriasis, acne and freckles. Hippocrates encouraged his fellow healers to use salts for their healing properties by immersing their patients in sea water. A Roman doctor by the name of Pedanius Dioscorides published his *De Materia Medica*, in which he recommends salt as an effective treatment for wounds, bites and problems with the digestion.

In 1750, British physician Richard Russell published a Latin dissertation *De Tabe Glandulari*, in which he recommended the use of sea water for the cure of enlarged lymphatic glands. Russell opened a practice in the seaside town of Brighton where he treated his patients with immersion in sea water and even the drinking of it (see page 43). Russell is credited with playing a major role in the mania for sea bathing and salt water cures in Britain during the second half of the 18th century.

As well as its medicinal properties, salt has long been prized for its cosmetic benefits. Cleopatra is said to have soaked in the mineral-rich waters of the Dead Sea, which she believed had mystical healing powers. She attributed her famed beauty to its waters. Salts were known to soften and smooth the skin, decreasing the appearance of fine lines.

The Role of Magnesium

Sea water is rich in magnesium and many people believe that being immersed in it for short periods of time while bathing at the beach allows your skin to absorb the magnesium you need.

Magnesium is the fourth most abundant mineral in the human body and every single cell needs magnesium to function. It is essential for strong bones and teeth, energy production and controlling blood sugar levels, blood pressure regulation, conducting nerve impulses, muscle contraction and normal heart rhythm.

Although we get most of our magnesium through the food we eat, it is not always well absorbed by the digestive track, and even more difficult to absorb in this way for those who are deficient in vitamin D, have poor gut bacteria or suffer from a number of other health conditions. We can, however, absorb magnesium through our skin and for those of us not able to bathe regularly in the ocean to top up our magnesium, there are some easy ways to supplement at home (see pages 130–5).

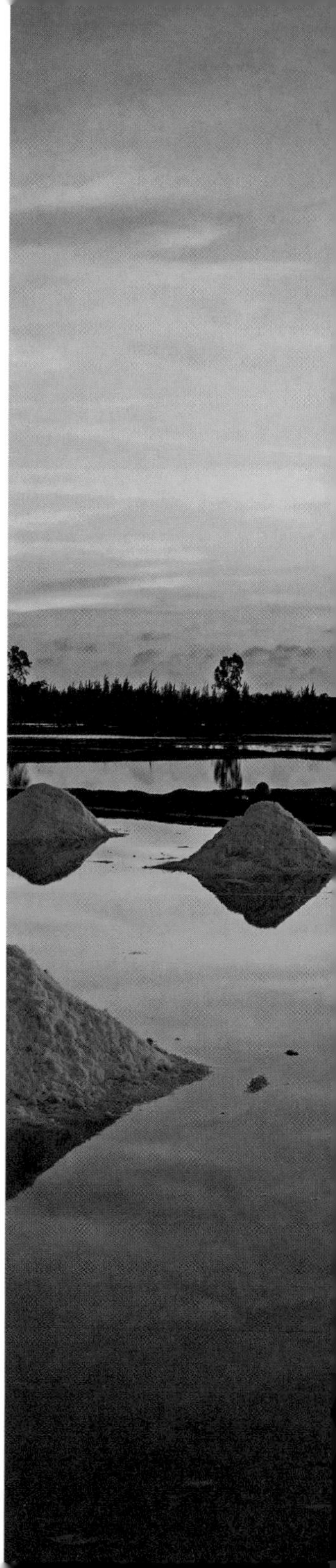

SALT BATHS, SPRAYS AND SCRUBS

Therapeutic and beauty products based around salt represent a huge industry and there are many ways to reap the benefits of salt and magnesium at home. While there are many commercial products available, it is easy to make your own, and you can be sure there are no artificial perfumes or other chemicals in them.

There are many different types of sea salt available, offering a range of possible benefits. Any of these salts can be used in the recipes on pages 132–5.

- **Epsom salts** – also known as magnesium sulphate, this is commonly used by athletes for soothing sore muscles and offers an inexpensive way to get the benefits of magnesium in a bath.
- **Dead Sea salt** – people have been flocking to bathe in the Dead Sea since classical times to treat skin conditions and improve their complexion. Dead Sea salt is said to contain 21 minerals including magnesium, potassium and calcium.
- **Red Alaea salt** – sea salt mixed with red Alaea volcanic clay which is said to have detoxifying properties, removing impurities under the skin. Native Hawaiians considered this clay to be a sacred, powerful healing tool and used it to treat broken bones, bug bites and burns.
- **Black lava sea salt** – sea salt infused with activated coconut-shell charcoal recommended for a detoxifying bath. Activated charcoal is said to attract skin oil, dirt and impurities, clearing acne and blemishes.

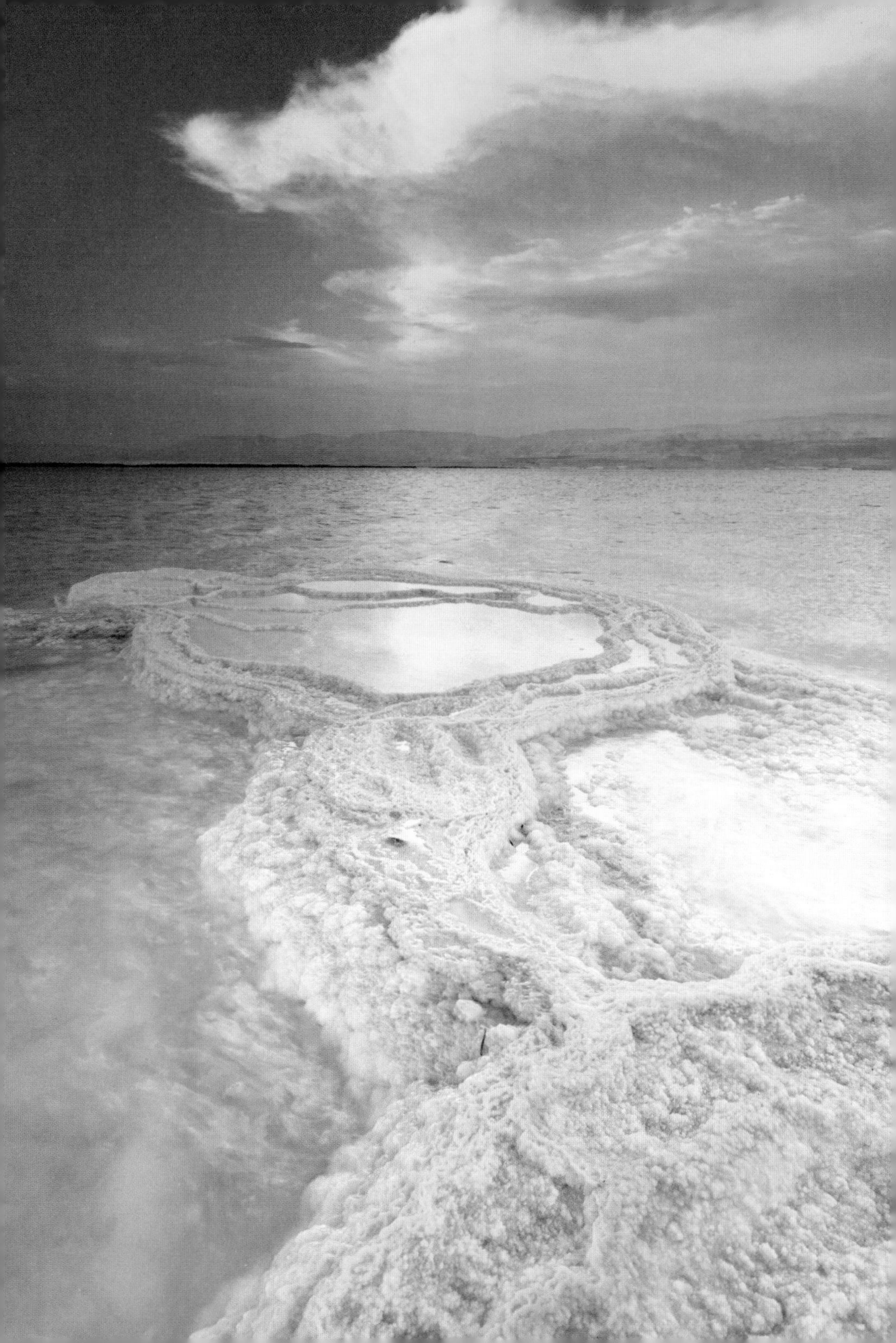

Sea Salt Spray

Many people notice an improvement in their complexion and a reduction in acne from the use of salt on the skin and this is a simple way to deliver it. The minerals in the salt can also help nourish skin. This spray leaves skin feeling refreshed and can be used as a facial toner or all over the body as a nourishing spray.

1 tablespoon sea salt
pinch of Epsom salts
240ml (8¾fl oz) boiled water
1–3 drops of essential oil, such as tea tree or lavender (optional)

Add the salts to the hot water, stir until dissolved then leave to cool. Add the essential oil, if using, and store in a spray bottle or glass jar. Apply to the skin daily by spraying or using a cotton pad.

Magnesium Oil

Although it is known as magnesium oil, this is actually a mixture of magnesium and water but it has a slightly greasy feeling on the skin like an oil. It is an efficient way to top up magnesium levels. It may cause a tingling sensation the first few times you use it, but this should soon fade.

125g (4½oz) magnesium chloride flakes
120ml (4 fl oz) boiled water

Add the magnesium chloride flakes to the hot water, stir until dissolved then leave to cool. Store in a spray bottle and apply daily to arms, legs and stomach. Leave on the skin to soak in, or rinse off after 20 minutes.

Magnesium Lavender Foot Scrub

This exfoliating and moisturizing scrub has a cooling sensation to ease dry, irritated skin. Liquid castile soap is a natural soap made from coconut and sunflower oils. It has a neutral pH that will not dry the skin.

60ml (4 tablespoons) olive oil or almond oil
1 teaspoon liquid castile soap
10–15 drops lavender essential oil
250g (9oz) Epsom salts or magnesium chloride flakes

Mix the oil, soap and essential oil until combined, then stir in the salt and store in an airtight jar. Use 1 teaspoon of the mixture as a foot scrub, working it into the soles of the feet, especially around areas of cracked or hard skin. Rinse after use.

SALT BATHS

Soothing salt baths are probably the easiest way to reap the benefits of salt water. They have been used for centuries to treat the following conditions:

- Aching muscles
- Stress
- Headaches
- Bad circulation
- Skin conditions such as acne and eczema
- Dry skin
- Respiratory problems
- Sleep problems
- Wounds and bruising

Salt can be used on its own in a warm bath, but other ingredients can be added to enhance the experience, including oils to aid skin hydration and essential oils for an aromatherapy experience.

Simple Bath Salts

These bath salts are ideal for use in a relaxing bedtime bath as lavender will help you sleep. However, if you have other favourite essential oils, feel free to use them instead, keeping quantities the same. Different oils have different therapeutic properties,[152] but most will engender a sense of wellbeing and relaxation.

2 tablespoons coconut or almond oil
10 drops peppermint essential oil
30 drops lavender essential oil
500g (1lb 2oz) Epsom salts
60g (2¼oz) Dead Sea salt (optional)

Mix the oil with the essential oils until well combined. Add the salts and mix again. Run a warm bath, add about 60g (2¼oz) of the bath salts and swirl around until dissolved. Soak for around 20 minutes. Store the remaining bath salts in an airtight jar.

Detox Bath Salts

These bath salts will sooth skin irritation and boost magnesium levels. As with any detox bath, you may feel lightheaded or very tired when you get out, so this one is best just before bed.

70ml (2½fl oz) apple cider vinegar
10 drops essential oil, such as lavender, thyme or rosewood
60g (2¼oz) sea salt
60g (2¼oz) Epsom salts

Run a warm bath, add all the ingredients and swirl around until dissolved. Soak for around 20 minutes.

FLOTATION THERAPY

People have been visiting the Dead Sea for thousands of years to float in its waters and benefit from the salts and minerals there. The high concentration of dissolved mineral salts in the water means the water is denser than the human body so we float. This effortless floating in salt-rich water is known to have a range of health benefits, and the same experience is recreated as a therapy all around the world.

Many spas offer flotation therapy in special pods designed to block out external distractions including sight, sound, tactile sensations and gravity. The pod contains a strong solution of Epsom salts, which is heated to skin temperature, as is the air in the pod, to remove all external stimulation.

Research shows that flotation therapy can lower levels of the stress hormone cortisol, lower blood pressure, improve wellbeing and enhance performance.[153] It is thought that flotation therapy combats stress in two ways. First, the magnesium in the water inhibits ACTH (adrenocorticotropin), the hormone that instructs the adrenal glands to release cortisol.[154] And secondly, magnesium improves sleep quality, which in turns leads to lower stress levels.[155]

Flotation therapy has also been shown to speed up recovery after a workout by lowering levels of lactic acid in the blood, which reduces overall muscle stiffness and pain.[156] Another study showed that flotation therapy improved the technical ability of musicians during jazz improvisation.[157]

Seaweed Therapies

Over the years, many studies have been conducted on the nutritional composition and health benefits of seaweeds, most of them concerning the use of seaweeds as foods or medicines. Some of this research has shown that seaweeds could play a role in the treatment or prevention of heart disease and some types of cancer, as well as improving thyroid and immune function, allergies and inflammation, and having antioxidant, antiviral and antibacterial qualities.[158]

Not surprisingly, the cosmetics industry has started to explore seaweeds as a cheap and sustainable source of natural ingredients for a wide range of products and therapies. We know seaweeds are bursting with nutrients – vitamins, minerals, proteins, starches and healthy fats – which are hugely beneficial when eaten, but many of these nutrients can also be absorbed through the skin. It seems that seaweeds can offer great benefits when applied as creams, lotions, face masks, body wraps and in warm baths.

There are now many ranges of skin-care products based around seaweed, including scrubs, exfoliators, face and body masks, moisturizers, face serums, hand creams, anti-inflammatory gels and sun-care products. Seaweeds boast so many beneficial ingredients that these products are designed to treat a variety of complaints, from dry skin, redness, eczema, psoriasis, acne, sun damage and dermatitis, to cellulite, premature ageing, fine lines and wrinkles, age spots and aching muscles. These products are known as "cosmeceuticals", a term coined for cosmetics that have pharmaceutical properties and can be used to treat certain medical conditions.

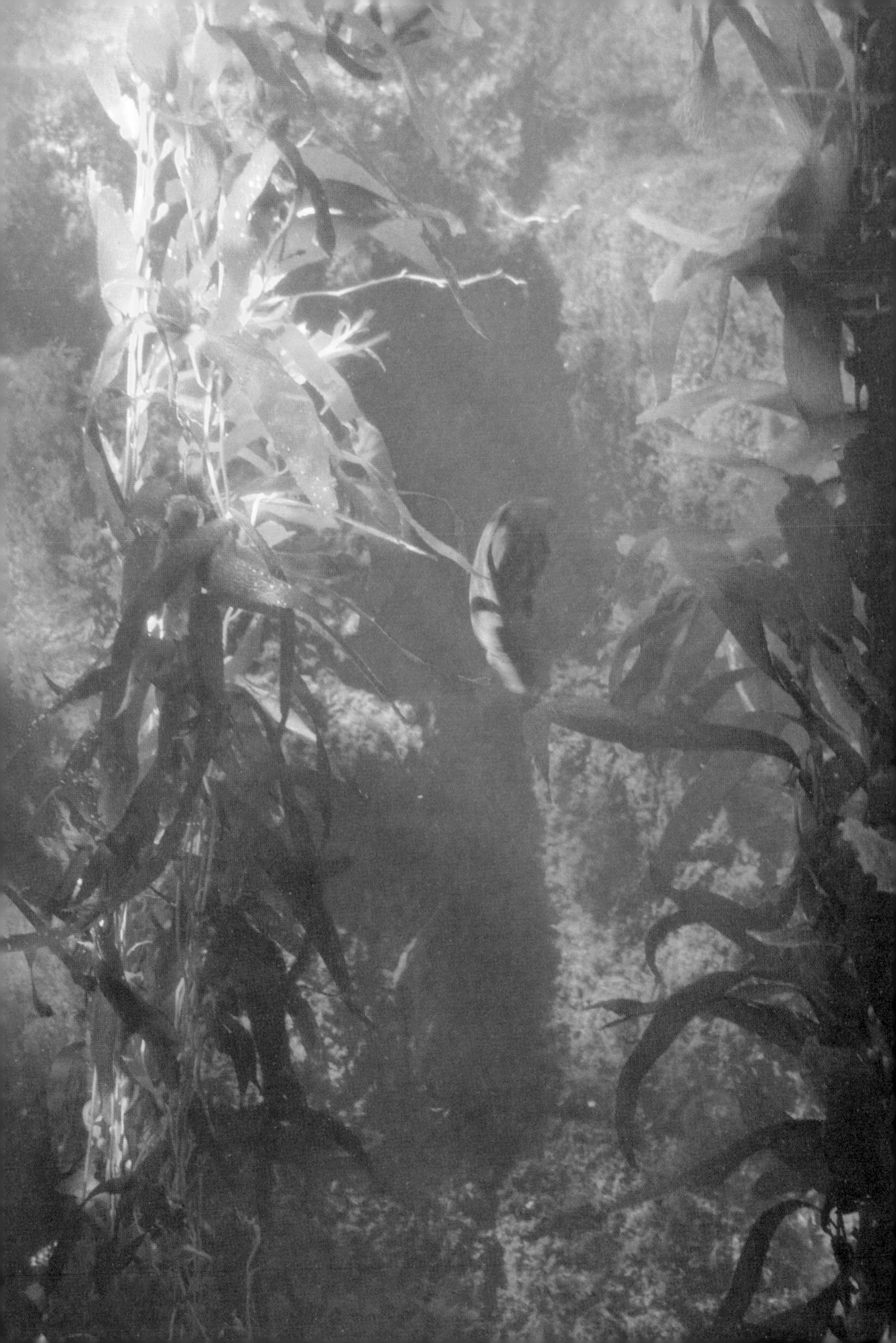

BENEFITS OF SEAWEED THERAPIES

Although some manufacturers of seaweed-based products make fairly exaggerated claims, research is showing some interesting findings:[159]

- Phlorotannins in brown seaweeds are being investigated for their potential to prevent damage from UV radiation and protect against skin cancers and premature aging.
- Some seaweeds, such as *Laminaria japonica*, have attracted great attention in the search for natural tyrosinase-inhibitor agents, which can lighten skin.
- Bioactive sesquiterpenes isolated from red and brown seaweeds have shown antibacterial and antiviral action and could be beneficial in fighting skin infections, including acne.[160]
- Phlorotannins from brown seaweeds can inhibit the activity of hyaluronidase, which is known to be involved in the allergic effects of dermatitis. The effect in one study was seven times stronger than that of DSCG (disodium cromoglycate), an active component in anti-allergic drugs.[161]
- Due to its high levels of phloroglucinol, the seaweed *Ecklonia cava* is used to treat allergic diseases in Asian countries such as Korea. Research has confirmed a potential anti-allergic mechanism.
- Phlorotannins from brown seaweeds are capable of inhibiting the release of histamine, which causes many of the symptoms of allergies, and may have a role in repairing skin damage from various allergens, which could be useful in the treatment of allergic conditions such as atopic dermatitis.
- Fucoidans – polysaccharides that are exclusively found in seaweeds – are being studied extensively for their possible antitumor, antiviral and anti-inflammatory activities. They may be used to prevent and treat the premature aging of skin through exposure to UV light and protect against the loss of elasticity.
- Moisturizing and hydration are essential to maintaining the elasticity of skin and protecting against environmental damage. Natural humectants in seaweeds can improve the skin's moisturizing ability and relieve dry skin conditions.
- Some peptides in seaweeds appear to reduce the appearance of fine wrinkles on the skin by strengthening components of the extracellular tissue matrix (ETM), such as collagen, hyaluronic acid and andelastin.

SEAWEED FACE MASKS

Making a seaweed face mask at home is an easy way to reap the benefits of seaweed to reduce the appearance of age spots, wrinkles, acne and excess pigmentation, while making skin tauter, smoother and better nourished. Seaweed face masks are suitable for any skin types – particularly mature skin – but avoid using them if you have allergies, very sensitive skin or large areas of broken skin.

Use good-quality powdered seaweed for these masks, which is readily available online. For the simplest mask, simply mix the seaweed to a paste with a little water, apply to the face and leave for 3–5 minutes before rinsing off. Apply a seaweed face mask no more than once a week.

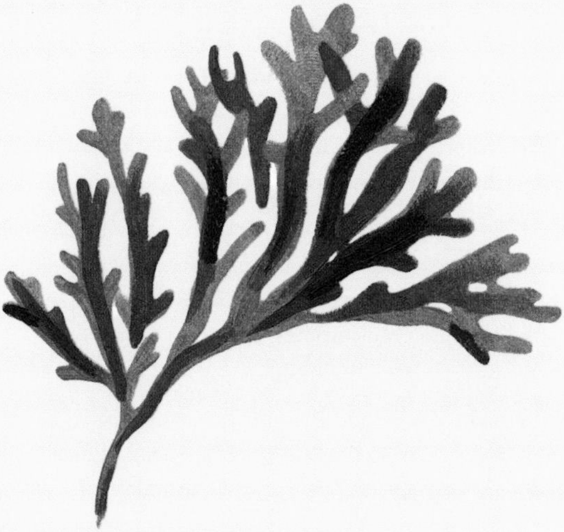

Seaweed and Honey Face Mask

Honey has antibacterial and soothing properties, making this mask particularly suitable for acne-prone skin.

1 tablespoon powdered seaweed
2 tablespoons warm water
1 teaspoon honey

Mix the seaweed and warm water in a bowl and leave for 1–1½ hours for the seaweed to absorb the water and swell up.

Place the mixture on a piece of clean muslin and squeeze gently over a bowl to collect all the liquid. Discard the seaweed.

Add the honey to the liquid and mix well. Use your fingertips to apply the mixture to your clean face and leave for 10 minutes. Wash off with clean, warm water.

Seaweed and Aloe Mask for Acne

Aloe vera has cooling and calming properties, making this mask great for soothing irritated skin.

1 tablespoon powdered seaweed
2 tablespoons warm water
1 tablespoon pure aloe vera gel

Mix the seaweed and warm water in a bowl and leave for 20 minutes.

Drain off any excess liquid and discard. Mix the aloe vera gel with the seaweed to form a paste. Use your fingertips to apply the mixture to your clean face and leave for 15 minutes. Wash off with clean, cool water.

BODY WRAPS

Seaweed body wraps work on the same principle as seaweed face masks, but they cover more of the body. These are very popular treatments in spas, but body wrap products are also available commercially and can be used at home. They are said to reduce fatty deposits by increasing metabolism, improve the appearance of cellulite and reduce fluid retention. Some people report losing an inch or two around the waist or thighs after the treatment, but this is a temporary loss due to the reduction in fluid retention.

If you have a wrap in a spa, nutrient-rich seaweed will be applied to all or part of your body, then you will be swaddled in a sheet, towels or thermal blanket and left to relax. The heat of the wrap will open your pores, relax your muscles and encourage you to sweat. Even if the inch loss is only temporary, you will certainly receive a boost of beneficial minerals and your skin will feel softer, smoother and hydrated.

SEAWEED BATHS

Another way to enjoy the therapeutic effects of seaweed is in a relaxing warm bath. This is another treatment offered in spas and retreat hotels. Dried seaweed, usually kelp, is simply placed in a bath of warm water, sometimes sea water, and the bather relaxes in the bath. In Ireland – a country that has long-since recognized the benefits of seaweeds for food and therapy – seaweed used to be known as the poor man's doctor and seaweed baths were used by generations to help them through the long winters.

As with other seaweed treatments, the beneficial vitamins and minerals from the seaweed are absorbed through the skin, but it seems that with a seaweed bath, the iodine can also enter the body by being inhaled in the steam from the bath. Iodine is essential for thyroid function, and thyroid hormones play a role in breaking down fat deposits in the body so it's possible that a seaweed bath could help reduce fatty deposits as well as offering all the skin benefits.

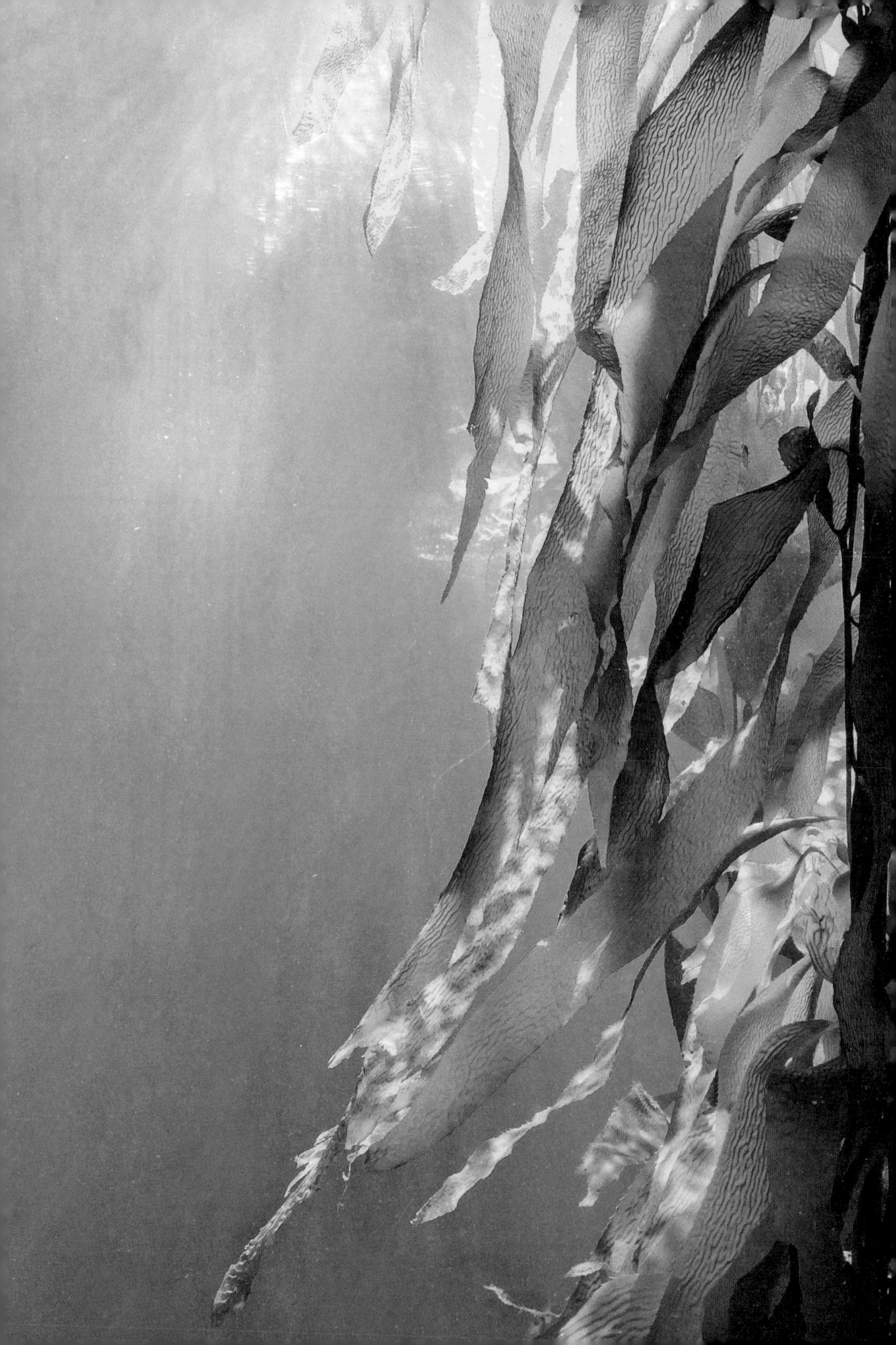

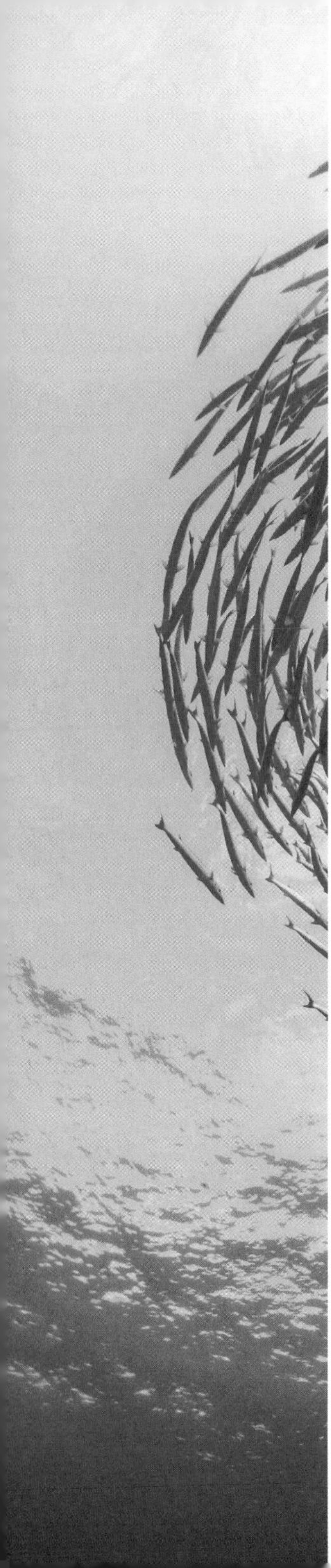

Bringing the Sea into Your Diet

We don't have to live near the sea to benefit from one of its greatest gifts – seafood. Seafood is simply one of the most nutritious foods we can put on our plates. But it's also delicious and hugely versatile – there are so many different varieties, which can be enjoyed in so many different ways.

Fish and seafood is low in calories, high in protein and rich in natural oils and other nutrients which benefit every part of our bodies. Here are some good reasons to include seafood in your diet.

- Seafood contains many of the minerals that are essential for good health, including iodine, zinc, selenium and potassium. These minerals support every system in our bodies and can help to protect us from cancers. Fish and shellfish also contain a range of vitamins, including vitamins A and D.
- Fish, particularly oily fish, is low in saturated fat and high in omega-3 fatty acids, which help lower cholesterol and reduce the risk of heart disease.
- Research suggests that people who eat plenty of fish and seafood are less likely to suffer from dementia and memory loss in later life, possibly because the brain is 60 per cent fat, much of it omega-3 fatty acids.
- DHA, an omega-3 fatty acid found in oily fish, has been linked to improvements in concentration among children, improved reading skills and a reduction in the incidence of attention deficit hyperactivity disorder (ADHD).
- Eating fish can help maintain good circulation and reduce the risk of thrombosis.
- Eating oil-rich fish regularly can help to protect against the effects of macular degeneration in later life, which causes eyesight to become blurred. Fish and shellfish also contain retinol, which boosts night vision.

- Eating fish regularly has been shown to help the symptoms of rheumatoid arthritis, a condition which causes the joints to swell. Recent research has also found a link between omega-3 fatty acids and the prevention of osteoarthritis.
- Seafood can relieve the symptoms of asthma in children, and may even be able to prevent it. Eating a lot of fish can also keep lungs stronger and healthier in later life.
- Fish is rich in protein, a building block of collagen, which helps to keep skin firm and elastic. The omega-3 fatty acids in fish help to protect skin from UV damage, and eating lots of fish can also help clear eczema and psoriasis.
- Research has shown links between low omega-3 levels and an increased risk of depression. This might be why the Japanese, with one of the most fish-rich diets in the world, have very low levels of depression.
- Fish oils can help prevent bowel diseases such as Crohn's disease and ulcerative colitis. There is also evidence to suggest that omega-3 may slow the progression of inflammatory bowel disease.

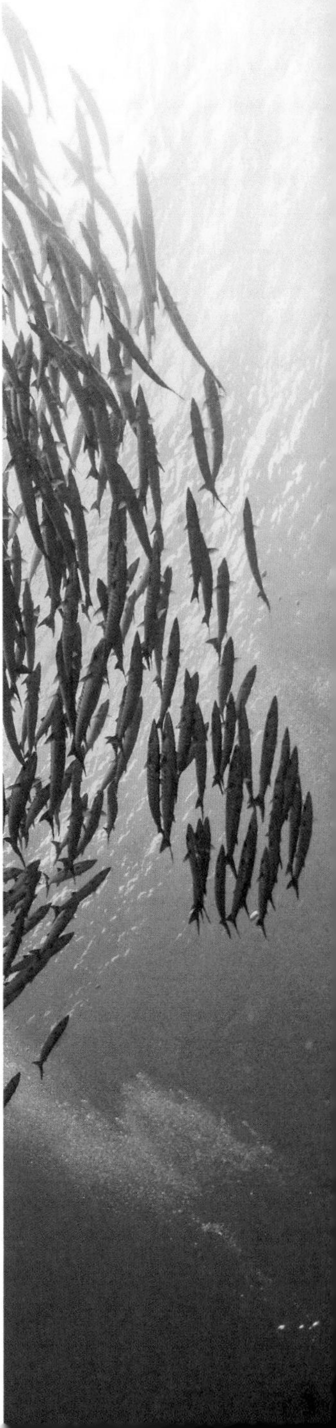

TYPES OF FISH

Different types of fish and shellfish provide different nutrients, so which should we be focusing on for the biggest health boost? The answer is all of them. All play an important role in a healthy diet and the more varieties you include in your diet, the greater the range of nutrients.

Oily Fish

Oily fish are rich in the all-important omega-3 fatty acids. They include salmon, mackerel, sardines, pilchards, fresh tuna, trout, whitebait, sprats and herring. Canned tuna does not count as an oily fish because the canning process reduces the amount of omega-3 fats to levels similar to those in white fish.

Some oily fish, such as whitebait, canned sardines, pilchards and canned salmon, contain bones that you can eat. They are good sources of calcium and phosphorus, and help to build strong bones and teeth.

White Fish

White fish include cod, haddock, plaice, pollock, sea bass, bream, monkfish, coley, dab, flounder, red mullet, whiting, gurnard and tilapia. They are low in fat and rich in protein, making them really healthy, low-fat alternatives to meat. These are really versatile fish which can be cooked in many different ways. They also contain omega-3 fats, but in lower quantities.

Shellfish

Shellfish include prawns, langoustines, lobster, crab, mussels, scallops, cockles and clams, squid and octopus. They are good sources of healthy low-fat protein and some types of shellfish – such as mussels, oysters, squid and crab – are also good sources of omega-3 fats, but they do not contain as much as oily fish.

HOW MUCH FISH SHOULD WE BE EATING?

Most sources recommend that a healthy diet should include at least two portions of fish each week, including one portion of oily fish.

But don't forget that frozen fish is just as nutritious as fresh and many different types are available. Canned sardines and mackerel can also make a delicious and hugely nutritious meal and have the added benefit of a dose of calcium.

Is There Anything to Avoid?

Some oily fish contain low levels of pollutants that can build up in the body. For this reason, it is best to have no more than four portions of oily fish a week (pregnant women, breastfeeding women and children should eat no more than two 140g/5oz portions). You can safely eat as much white fish as you like, apart from sea bass, bream, huss, turbot and halibut, which can contain similar levels of pollutants as oily fish.

Seafood is a great source of healthy protein during pregnancy and offers many benefits to a developing foetus. Studies have shown that children whose mothers ate fish during pregnancy had a higher intelligence quotient (IQ) than those whose mothers didn't.

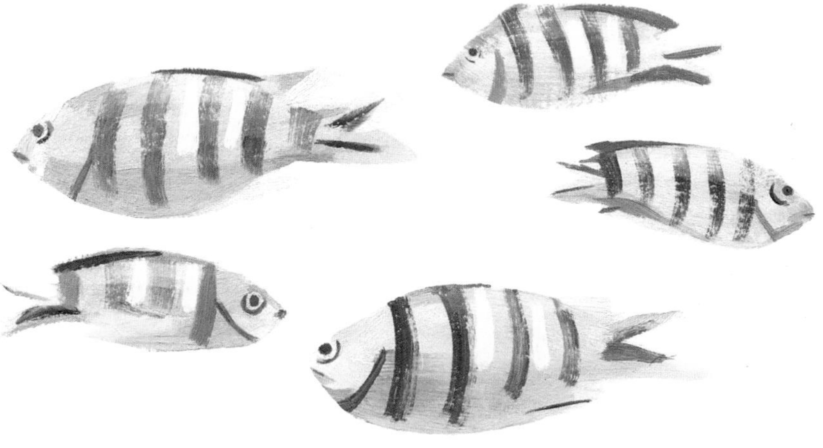

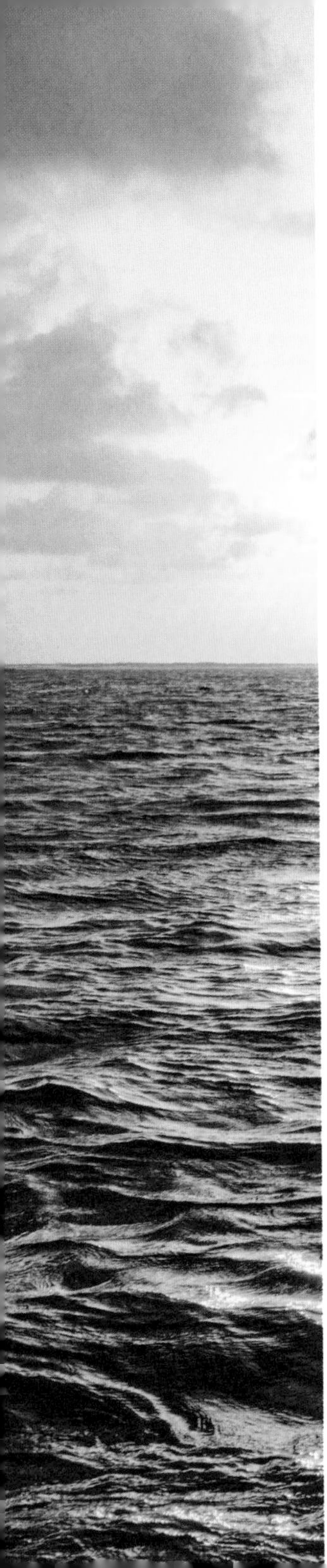

WHAT TO LOOK FOR WHEN BUYING FISH

Seafood is available to buy fresh, frozen, cured, canned or smoked. When buying frozen seafood, check it is frozen solid with no signs of partial thawing. Make sure that packaging is intact and there is no sign of freezer burn. Here's what to look for with fresh fish.

Whole Fish

- The eyes should be bright and not sunken.
- The skin should be shiny, moist and glossy with a coating of clear slime.
- You should notice a pleasant fresh aroma or none at all.
- The gills should be bright red, not brown or grey.

Fish Fillets

- The flesh should be moist with a glossy sheen; avoid any that look dry or dull.
- The fish should be firm and the bands of muscle should be tightly joined together.
- Fillets should have a fresh smell of the sea, or no smell at all.

Smoked Fish

- Smoked fish should look glossy.
- The flesh should be firm and plump.
- Smoked fish should have a fresh smoky aroma.

Shellfish

- Mussels, clams and oysters, if sold live, should have shells which are tightly closed without any gaps or cracks.

- Lobsters and crabs can be bought live or cooked. Either way they should be heavy for their size and all the legs should be attached and tight.
- Prawns, either raw or cooked, should have dry intact shells. If sold shelled, they should smell sweet and pleasant.
- Scallops can be sold raw in the shell – if they are, it doesn't matter if the shells are open. The flesh should be bright white and they should smell sweet.
- Squid and octopus should smell sweet and the flesh should be white and moist.

SUSTAINABILITY

Seafood is one of the world's most valuable resources. More and more, fishers are using good practices to maintain fish stocks and to help protect the marine environment. When seafood is caught or farmed in a way that allows stocks to replenish and does not cause unnecessary damage to other marine life, that seafood can be called "sustainable".

To ensure stocks are able to replenish themselves, choose from as wide a range of different species as possible. If we eat only a few kinds of fish, then stocks fall due to overfishing, which endangers the future supply of the fish and can cause damage to the environment it lives in. It is our responsibility to ensure that the seafood we eat comes from these well-managed and sustainable sources, so try to find out where your seafood was sourced before you buy it. For more information, see pages 157–8.

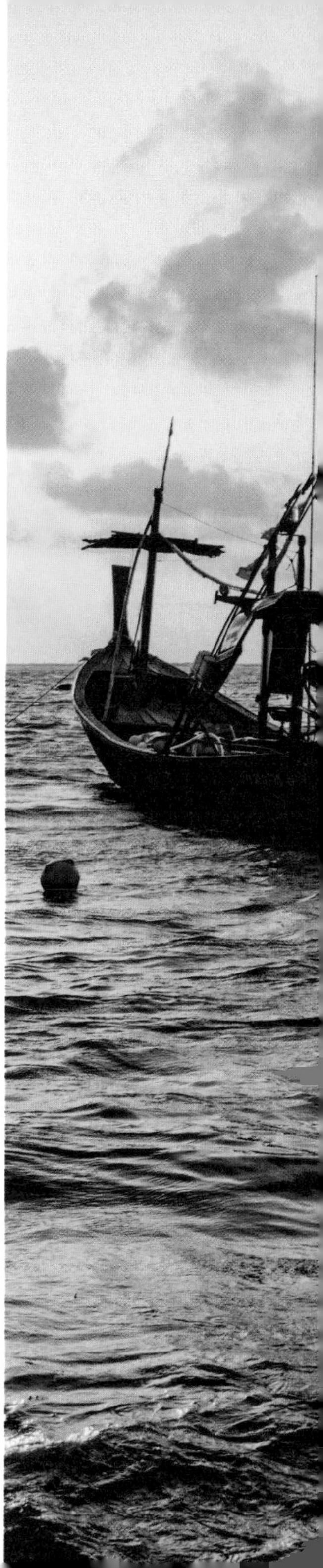

EDIBLE SEAWEEDS

Most of us are familiar with seaweed in our sushi and miso soup but probably don't realize that it packs a serious nutritional punch. Seaweed is bursting with antioxidants, vitamins and minerals and there are thought to be over 10,000 different species in the world, all varying in nutritional content and flavour.

Despite its recent popularity and superfood status, seaweed has been eaten all over the world for thousands of years, most notably in Japanese, Korean and Chinese cuisines. In parts of Europe, seaweeds also have a long history, in ancient medicine and folklore as well as in the kitchen.

Nutritional Benefits

The Japanese have one of the highest life expectancies in the world, and one significant dietary habit is their regular consumption of seaweeds. Seaweeds contain molecules known as fucoidans, which could be responsible for these impressive health benefits, contributing not just to longevity, but to immunity, cardiovascular function[162] and cancer prevention.[163] In 2011, a review of 100 studies on the benefits of seaweeds found that they may be used to help lower blood pressure and promote heart health.[164]

Seaweeds are much more nutrient-dense than any land vegetables. They contain a rich supply of minerals, most notably calcium, copper, iodine, magnesium, zinc and iron. They are also rich in protein, fibre and vitamins, especially vitamin K and folic acid, while being low in fat. Because of this impressive nutritional profile, seaweeds are thought to help the body fight illness and disease in many ways. Unlike land plants, seaweeds contain omega-3 fats (see pages 144–5), so seaweed or algae oil can be a reliable source of omega-3 for vegetarians and they are also one of the few vegetable sources of vitamin B^{12}.

Safety Warning

Such high concentrations of some of the nutrients can be a problem for some people. For example, too much vitamin K can interfere with blood-thinning medications, while too much potassium can be a problem for those with kidney disease. The high levels of iodine make seaweeds beneficial for thyroid health, but too much iodine can be detrimental. If you have any concerns, speak to your doctor.

Types of Seaweed and How to Use Them

If you live near an Asian supermarket, you may be able to find fresh seaweed. If not, many types of dried seaweeds are available in supermarkets, health food shops and online. Thicker dried seaweeds should be soaked in hot water and rinsed before use.

- Dried seaweed flakes or granules can be sprinkled over many foods, rather like seasoning, imparting a lovely salty, savoury flavour. Try them with rice dishes, fresh fish, soups and salads.
- Kombu is a brown kelp with a strong umami flavour. It is used to make dashi soup stock and can be added to stews or enjoyed in salads.
- Arame is another species of kelp which comes in dark brown strands. It has a mild sweet flavour and firm texture, and can be added to soups, stews, rice dishes and even baked goods.
- Kelp noodles are simply strands of raw kelp. They are a nutritious and gluten-free alternative to noodles, both low in calories and rich in calcium.
- Wakame has soft green fronds with a subtle sweet flavour and satiny texture. It is most famous as the seaweed found in miso soup but also makes a great salad ingredient.
- Dulse is a red seaweed with a softer, chewy texture. It is often dried and eaten as a healthy snack, while in Ireland it is baked in soda bread.
- Nori is shredded and dried into sheets to wrap sushi, or can be enjoyed as a savoury snack. It is also used to flavour noodle dishes and soups.
- Laver is a red seaweed which grows in delicate, soft sheets. It is widely used in China, Japan and Korea, and in Wales it is made into laverbread, a thick paste served as a vegetable or sauce.
- Most types of seaweed can be served as a Japanese salad, dressed with rice vinegar and sesame oil.

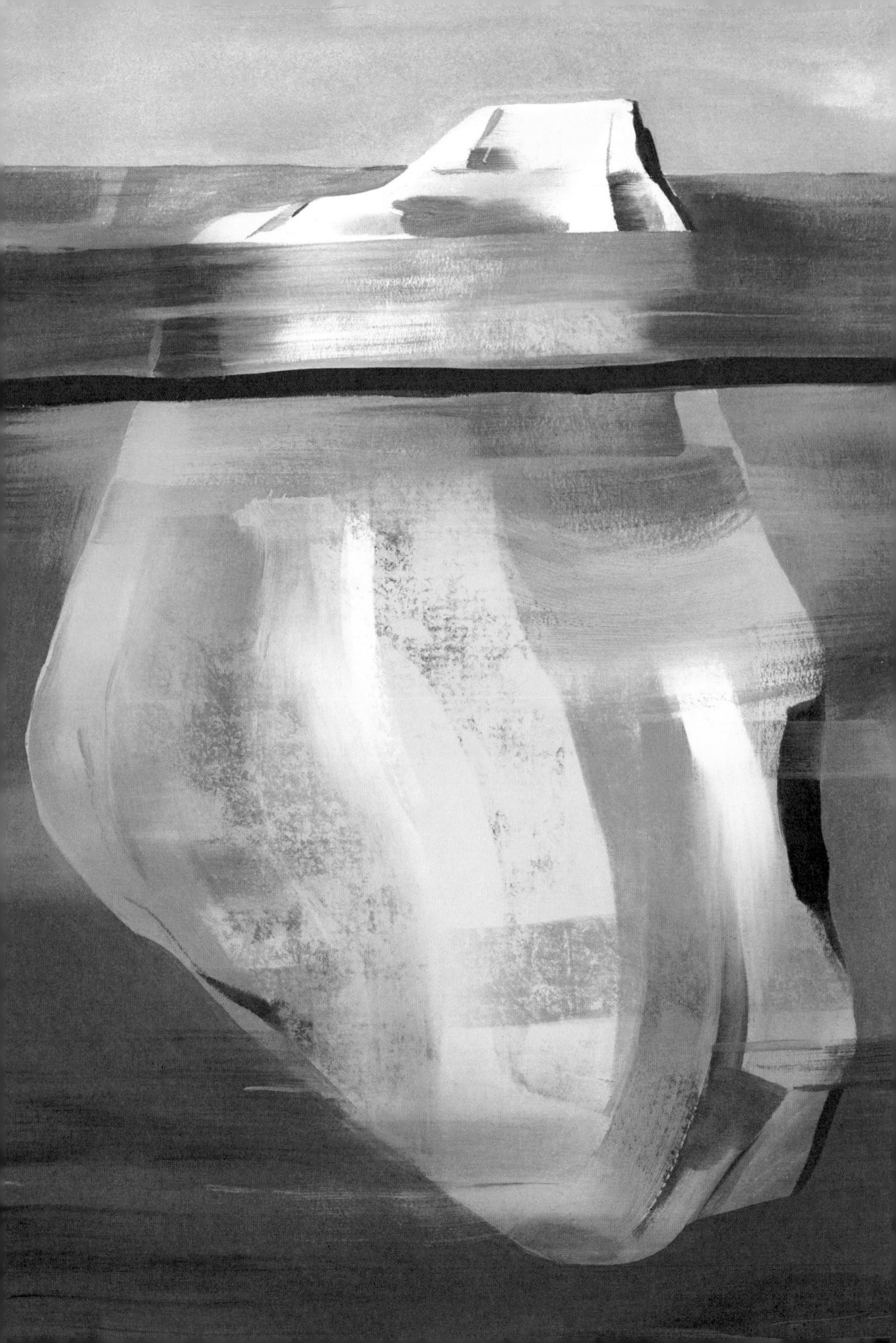

CHAPTER 6

Taking Care of the Oceans So They Take Care of Us

"There must be something strangely sacred in salt. It is in our tears and in the sea."

— Kahlil Gibran

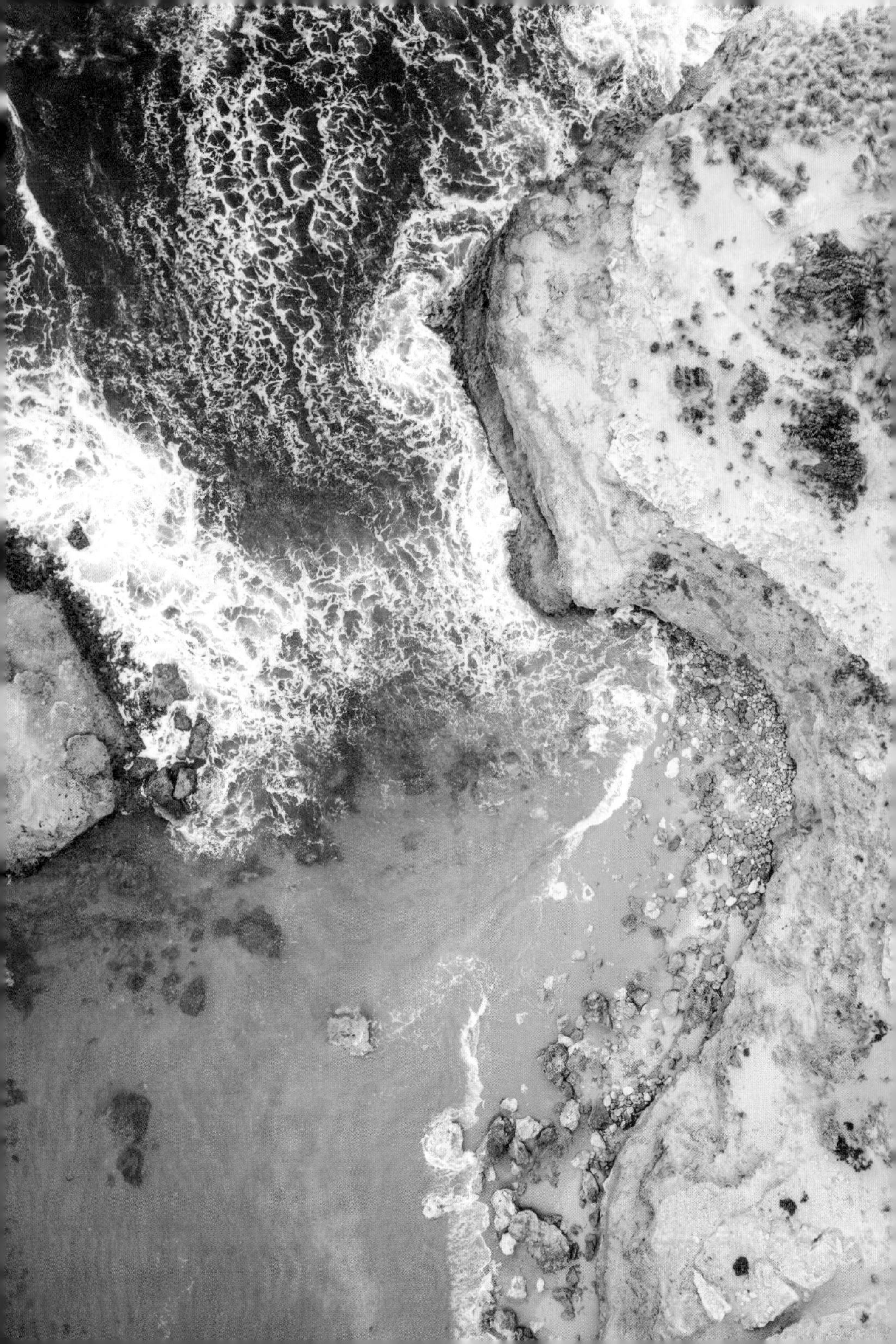

Throughout this book we have seen the amazing effects that the sea has on our physical and mental health and wellbeing. The ocean provides food and medicines, supports livelihoods, enables trade and commerce, promotes physical activity, offers opportunities for leisure, recreation and social interaction, creates a space for relaxation and contemplation, helps alleviate stress, is a source of beauty and inspiration, and is culturally and spiritually important.

Even the physical coastline itself is critical in helping to protect and support the health and wellbeing of millions of people globally, as intertidal habitats and coastal features – such as mangroves, reef systems and salt marshes – absorb wave energy and buffer the effects of sea level rise and increasing storms.[70]

We have seen how the sea and associated habitats are vital for our health and wellbeing, as well as being essential for the health of the whole planet. Unfortunately, however, these precious systems are under threat. Many factors are adversely affecting the health of our oceans and there is a growing consensus that many of these factors are a result of human activities, especially through the increased emission of greenhouse gases, such as carbon dioxide.[165] While factors such as climate change, overfishing and pollution all affect the health of the oceans, often human health and wellbeing is also impacted as a result.

Climate Change

The use of fossil fuels since the Industrial Revolution, and other human activities – such as deforestation and intensive livestock farming – have increased the level of greenhouse gases, such as carbon dioxide (CO_2), in the atmosphere. Greenhouse gases in the atmosphere trap heat radiating from the Earth (the "greenhouse effect"). The resulting rise in the Earth's surface temperature causes global warming and climate change.

Although geological evidence indicates that there have been natural changes to the climate in the past, the changes that we are experiencing now are occurring at an unprecedented rate. There is concern, therefore, that the biodiversity on the planet could be threatened, as species may not be able to adapt to these rapid changes quickly enough.[166]

The oceans absorb much of the excess CO_2, which has altered their pH, making them more acidic. This process of ocean acidification can adversely affect calcareous marine organisms, such as corals and molluscs, by making their skeletons less robust.[165] Increased concentrations of CO_2 in the atmosphere also affect temperatures. Global warming has been linked to changes in the life cycles, distribution and migration of animals on land, and in the sea.

Higher sea temperatures are particularly associated with coral bleaching, which is the expulsion of the corals' symbiotic algae (zooxanthellae) that can lead to coral die-off. Higher temperatures are also associated with melting sea ice which may pose other threats, such as flooding, which affect low-lying coastal ecosystems, as well as the homes and livelihoods of people who live along the coast.[165]

Overfishing and Destructive Fishing Practices

One of the greatest ecological threats facing the oceans is overfishing.[167] Fish and shellfish are an important source of protein yet the demands of an increasing human population, together with technological developments in the fishing industry, has led to overfishing and a rapid decrease in the populations of many fish species. Global fishing fleets are now so large and technically advanced that they are able to catch far more fish than the oceans can realistically provide. Many areas have been overfished, resulting in collapsing fish stocks as too few mature fish are left to breed and maintain the population.

Furthermore, many fishing methods – while effective – are extremely destructive. Bottom trawling for fish that live on or near the seabed, and dredging (for example for scallops and oysters), can ravage seabed habitats and communities, resulting in damage that can take the ecosystem years to recover from. Dynamite fishing – using dynamite to stun or kill fish, making them easier to collect – is another destructive fishing method. The explosions damage the habitat (including coral reefs) and the species they support, and also place fishers in danger.

Bycatch – the unintended capture of non-target species – is another problem. Sea turtles, dolphins, juvenile fish and other non-target species that are landed with the intended fish catch are subsequently discarded, usually dead or dying. The deliberate targeting of certain other species can also be a problem. For instance, tens of millions of oceanic sharks are caught each year in a largely unregulated industry.[167] Sharks are primarily caught for their fins and often returned to the water still alive where, unable to swim, they sink to the bottom and suffocate or are eaten by predators. It is also highly likely that the removal of so many top predators from the environment will affect the delicate balance of ecosystems.

FISH FARMING

The farming of aquatic species (aquaculture), as an alternative to catching them from the wild, can also be problematic. For instance, some species (such as salmon and prawns) are carnivorous and therefore require a huge supply of wild-caught fish to feed on, in the form of fish pellets. Furthermore, keeping large numbers of animals in confined areas along the coast, particularly in wetlands and mangroves, can negatively affect the marine environment and its wild populations: nursery habitats can be destroyed, large volumes of nutrients and waste can degrade the environment, any imported disease may spread to wild fish, and exotic species may escape, breed and multiply, potentially causing a negative effect on local populations and wild species.[168]

While the above practices are clearly damaging for marine ecosystems, the collapse of fish stocks through unsustainable fishing practices are also likely to affect the wellbeing of families and local communities by negatively impacting on their livelihoods and health.

Pollution

Pollution comes in many forms – air, water, soil, light, sound, thermal, radioactive – and many of these can adversely affect marine ecosystems.

CHEMICAL POLLUTANTS

Agricultural run-off, particularly during periods of heavy rain, can wash pesticides and excess nutrients (such as nitrogen and phosphorous) into rivers, estuaries and the oceans. Excessive nutrients can cause algae and other phytoplankton to proliferate (a process known as eutrophication), and can result in the formation of algal blooms, some of which may be toxic. Harmful algal blooms (HABs) can affect both wildlife and humans, who may consume the fish and shellfish that have been affected by HAB toxins. Eutrophication can create areas of low oxygen which, if extreme, can generate "dead zones" in the sea.[4] Pesticide residues can persist in the environment and accumulate within the food chain, negatively affecting the health of aquatic organisms.

Other chemical substances – such as polycyclic aromatic hydrocarbons (PAHs), heavy metals like methyl mercury, and pharmaceuticals such as synthetic hormones – can also enter the marine environment. Some substances that contaminate waterways and the oceans can disrupt the endocrine system of aquatic organisms. These are the glands responsible for secreting hormones and other products into the blood. These endocrine-disrupting chemicals (EDCs) can be synthetic (such as oral contraceptives, detergents and pesticides), or natural (such as human and animal hormones that are found in sewage and farming run-off), and can adversely affect the health of an organism or its offspring in a variety of ways. For example, changes that can negatively impact wild populations include instances of feminized male fish, masculinized female gastropod molluscs, disrupted development of fish embryos, and the increased incidence of disease and tumour in flatfish.[169]

Contaminants can not only affect marine life but also the humans who eat contaminated food.[4] One of the most well-known cases of heavy metal poisoning occurred in Japan. First noticed in the Japanese city of Minamata, seafood contaminated with methyl mercury from industrial waste water has been responsible for the illness and death of thousands of people in Japan since the 1950s.

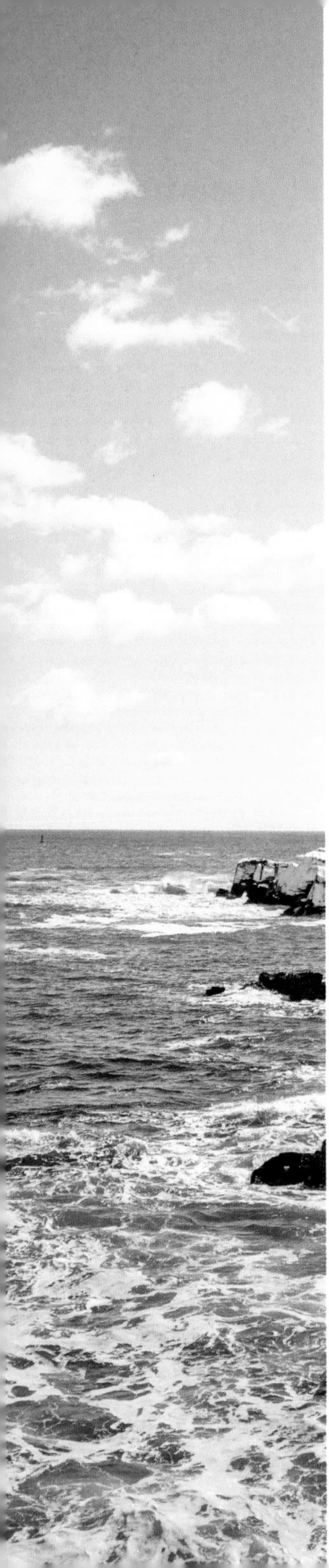

SEWAGE

Bacteria and viruses from both animals and human sources can affect water quality for recreational and commercial use. Bathing in affected water brings human health risks through the contraction of infections and illnesses (such as ear infections and gastroenteritis), and seafood can become contaminated resulting in seafood poisoning.[4] Even the perception of poor water quality can prevent people from engaging with the marine environment,[170] thus stopping them from gaining the benefits of enhanced wellbeing that visits to the sea can bring.

OIL SPILLS

Over the years, oil spills have damaged marine ecosystems. Numerous oil spills around the world have included both high-profile spills from oil rigs and production platforms (such as the Deepwater Horizon in the Gulf of Mexico in 2010), and supertanker accidents (such as the Exxon Valdez in the Persian Gulf in 1991 and the Amoco Cadiz in France in 1978). These spills have all contaminated hundreds of square miles of sea and coastline, and killed hundreds of thousands of animals, including sea birds, sea otters, whales and fish. People have also lost their livelihoods and sometimes their lives in these disasters.

LIGHT AND NOISE POLLUTION

Marine animals can be affected by light and noise pollution. Marine turtles, for instance, rely on light cues, and artificial lighting close to nesting sites can disorientate them.[171] The presence of night lighting can affect the nesting behaviour of female turtles by deterring them from visiting nesting beaches. Turtle hatchlings, who use moonlight reflected on the water as a visual cue to head towards the ocean, can head towards sources of artificial lighting instead.[172]

For other species, noise can cause confusion. Whales and dolphins navigate, communicate and locate their food using sounds. Ocean noise from boat traffic, seismic surveys or the use of sonar can adversely affect these abilities, placing them in danger of stranding and death.[173]

MARINE LITTER

Of all the pollution issues, marine litter is currently one of the most topical. Manmade debris is found throughout the marine environment, from the poles to the equator, along shorelines and from the surface of the sea to the ocean depths.[174] Marine debris is defined as any solid material that is processed or manufactured and that subsequently ends up in the marine or coastal environment. Items may be deliberately disposed of, discarded, abandoned or unintentionally lost, either on land or at sea.

Marine litter items may include glass, rubber, wood or metal, but most marine litter is made of plastic. While plastic may be considered a versatile and useful material, its "useful" properties, such as its durability, can make it resistant to degradation. As a result, it is extremely persistent and prevalent throughout the oceans. Since the 1960s, plastic production has increased from 5 million tonnes to 280 million tonnes in 2011, although we cannot be certain exactly how much of this has found its way into the oceans.[174]

The impact of marine debris on marine life is of particular concern and is thought to be one of the major perceived threats to marine biodiversity. Marine debris is thought to affect the environments in four key ways:[174]

- It can become a source of entanglement and ingestion.
- It can disperse species to other areas ("rafting").
- It can impact habitat community structures.
- It can provide a new habitat for colonization.

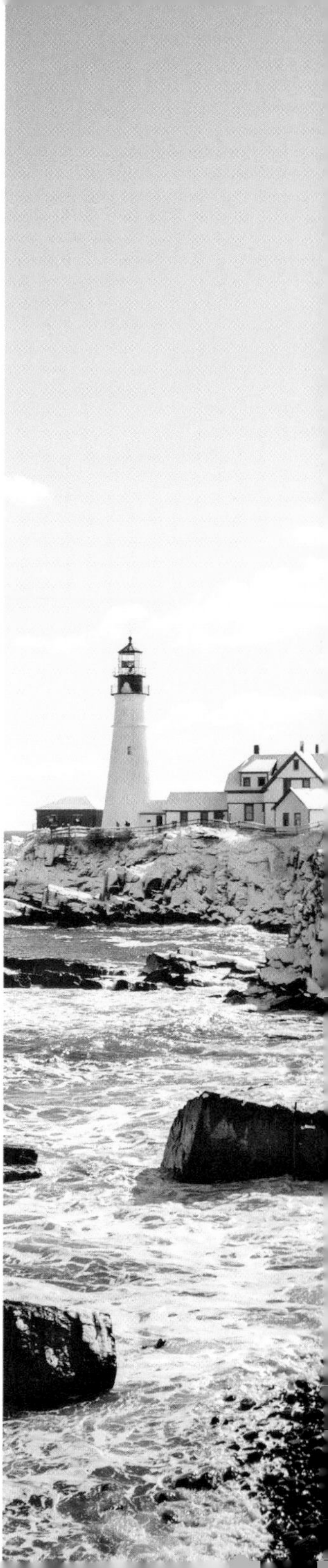

THE IMPACT OF MARINE DEBRIS

One well-known issue associated with marine debris is that of entanglement and ingestion. Although exact numbers can never be known, studies have reported that almost 400 species and over 44,000 animals have encountered marine debris, and fatalities have been recorded for many species. Most encounters involved plastic debris with many animals becoming entangled in plastic rope and netting or ingesting plastic fragments. All known species of sea turtle and over 50 per cent of marine mammal and sea bird species have been affected by marine debris, as well as numerous other species.

Around 17 per cent of species affected were those most at risk of extinction according to the IUCN Red List of Threatened Species. These include the giant manta ray, the great white shark, many seabird species (such as albatross, petrel and shearwater species) and six of the seven species of sea turtle, including Kemp's ridley and hawksbill sea turtles, both of which are classified as "Critically Endangered".[174] Small plastic particles called "microplastics" have also been found in mussels and oysters grown for human consumption, although the effects on our health and wellbeing are currently unknown.[175]

Habitats, such as coral reefs, can be physically damaged by marine debris. For instance, lost fishing gear can scrape and rub against sponges and corals, and the resulting tissue abrasion can cause partial or total mortality.

Marine ecosystems can also be impacted by the colonization of non-native species which attach themselves to marine debris and become transported to areas in which they do not usually live. These invasive species can upset the balance of existing ecosystems, causing unwanted changes to marine habitats and communities.

Once more, there is potential for marine debris to affect human health and wellbeing. As marine debris can threaten biodiversity, a degraded and less biodiverse environment is likely to negatively impact on human health and wellbeing, as coastal environments perceived to have a greater diversity and abundance of marine life are thought to offer greater emotional and cognitive restoration potential.[126]

The visual presence of marine debris on our beaches can also have an effect. A photo study in which participants rated different beach scenes, with and without litter, found that the presence of litter could undermine restorative benefits.[141] Interestingly, in this study, people differentiated between different litter types, rating "public litter" such as discarded plastic bottles as being more detrimental to psychological wellbeing than litter perceived to have originated from the fishing industry (such as remnants of old rope).

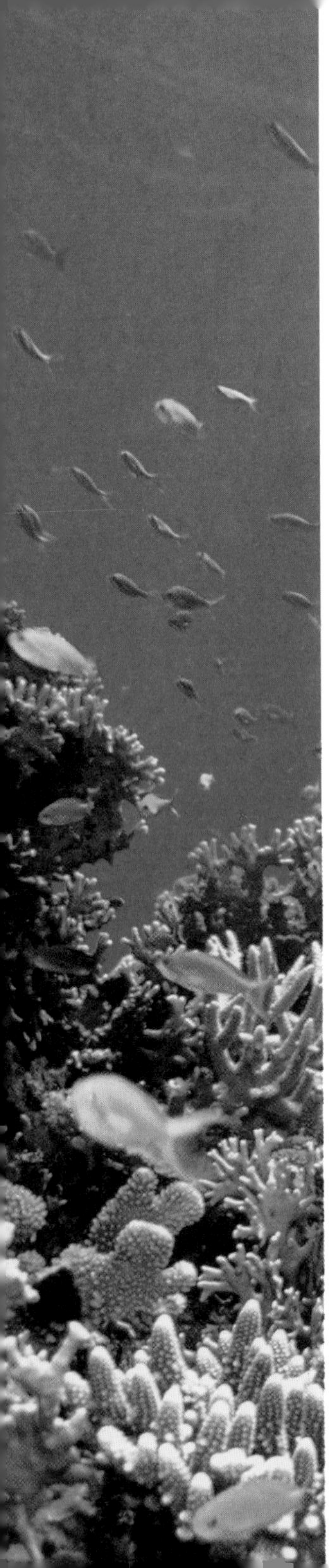

Coastal and Off-shore Development

Sandy beaches, locations we treasure for their aesthetic beauty, as well for relaxation, recreation and leisure, can be impacted by human activity. While storms have always naturally altered the topography of the coastline, the increasing number of extreme weather events and sea level rise, linked to climate change, is exacerbating the situation. Coastal development (for example expansion of existing cities and new locations for tourism) is adding to the problem. Altering the coast can increase erosion and therefore increase the likelihood of flooding and damage during storm surges. Poorly planned coastal zone areas can also increase litter and other forms of pollution in the water and along the coast, increase the incidents of industrial and agricultural contamination, and increase pollution associated with additional boat traffic.

Once again, these processes can impact on human health. For example, the popularity of a "home by the sea" may result in an increase in second-home ownership. This could have detrimental effects on the health and wellbeing of the local community. Local people may no longer be able to afford to purchase a property in their home town and may before forced to move away. For those who remain, community life may suffer if local facilities, such as shops and libraries, close through lack of year-round support.

Aggregate Extraction and Other Mining Activities

One of the biggest pressures on our beaches and seabeds is the removal of sand and gravel for the construction industry and for beach replenishment schemes elsewhere along the coast.[176] The construction industry around the world is booming and a global shortage of material is possible.[176] Although the construction industry provides employment (and is therefore beneficial to human health), it can also have adverse effects on ecosystems and those who rely on them. Sand-mining can increase the vulnerability of coastal regions to storm and tsunami events[4, 176] and reduce the availability of nursery grounds for juvenile fish. These in turn can negatively affect local people who rely on fishing and other industries for their livelihoods.

Aggregate extraction can also affect the marine environment: the composition of the sea substrate may change, species may become smothered, and community structure may be altered, perhaps reducing species richness and abundance.[177]

Mining of a different sort – coal mining – may also pose a threat to the oceans. A proposed coal mine in Queensland, Australia, and its associated infrastructure changes, could significantly impact coral reefs. It is suggested that the mine would significantly contribute to greenhouse gases, and dredging activities designed to enlarge the port may block sunlight, effectively starving the corals and adding to water pollution via increased shipping.[178]

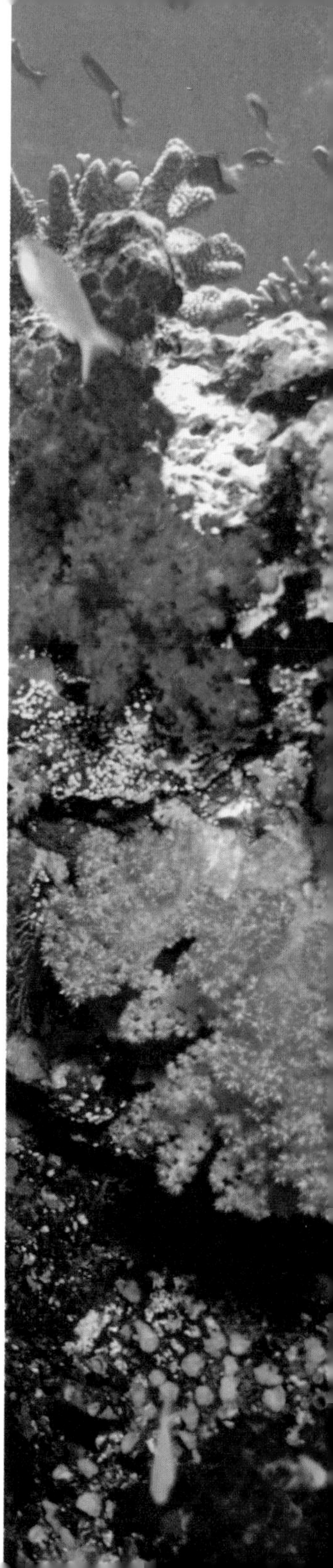

What Are the Solutions?

All in all, the pressures on our oceans tend to paint a gloomy picture. So is there anything that can be done? Thankfully, the answer is "Yes!". Scientists, industry, governments and non-governmental organizations (NGOs) are already working hard to help address some of these crucial issues: the complex interactions between living organisms and the non-living (chemical, physical) aspects of ecosystems are being studied; new products and techniques are being developed; more rigorous legislation is being implemented; and communities around the world are being educated, encouraged and supported in their efforts to conserve their local biodiversity and natural resources.

There is, however, also a lot that we, as individuals, can do to help look after our oceans – and, indeed, the planet as a whole. No individual action is too small not to make a difference – and collectively, we are even more powerful, and we can make a difference, however desperate the situation may seem. Throughout our evolution, our physical and mental health and wellbeing has benefitted from our positive interactions with the oceans. However, we humans, as a species, are harming this precious resource and the other species that live within it. We must therefore do all we can to protect the oceans, not simply for our benefit, but for the benefit of our planet and future generations.

WHAT CAN WE DO AROUND THE HOME?

Save Energy

- Turn off lights and appliances when you are not using them, and don't leave appliances on stand by.
- Buy energy-efficient appliances.
- Use energy-saving light bulbs.
- Turn down your thermostat by 1°C.
- Use an energy-monitoring device in your home.
- Ensure your home is adequately insulated and draft-proofed – check windows, doors, loft hatches.
- Use the economy setting when possible.
- Buy products that require less energy to produce.
- Consider solar energy.

Reduce Water Consumption

- Install water-efficient toilets, taps and shower heads.
- Turn off taps while brushing your teeth or washing your face.
- Have a shower instead of a bath.
- Repair any leaking taps and toilets.
- Ensure that there is a full load for the washing machine or dishwasher (this also helps with energy use).

Dispose of Waste Responsibly

- Only flush toilet paper (and human waste) down the toilet. Don't use the toilet as an extra rubbish bin – items like sanitary products, cotton buds, dental floss, "disposable" wipes, cigarette butts, grease, paint, food

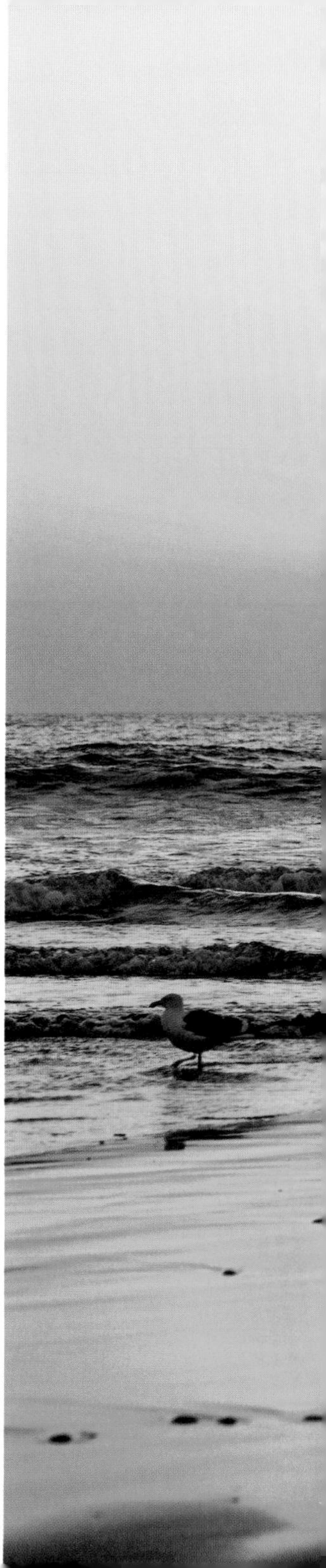

and old medication can damage wastewater treatment centres and cause environmental pollution. Also, less flushing means less water used.

- Dispose of hazardous materials properly – don't throw used motor oil down the drain.
- If you are thinking about buying a product you are unlikely to use very much, considering borrowing it from someone else. Look for a "Borrow, don't buy" scheme near you or consider setting up a scheme for people in your local area.
- If an electrical item or gadget no longer works, it may just need fixing rather than being thrown away. Attending a community Repair Café may help you get your item fixed for free.
- Put a "No Junk Mail" sign on your door.
- Buy products with less – or no – packaging.
- Find alternatives to food wrap – store food in reusable storage containers, use bowls with lids or cover with a reusable silicone lid.
- Thoroughly wash items before recycling – dirty items are less likely to be recycled.
- Consider if an item can be used for another purpose before throwing it away. Jars, boxes and other containers can be used for storage. Old wrapping paper, sweet wrappers, yogurt pots and pieces of ribbon can be used for art and craft activities. Be creative!
- Recycle old clothes, toys and books at your local charity shop. There is a good chance that someone else could put them to good use – and the charity will benefit from the extra income.

In the Garden

- To help reduce water usage, choose drought-resistant plants and mulch the soil to reduce evaporation.
- If you do need to water the plants, install a water butt to capture rainwater. Use sprinklers, garden hoses and pressure washers sparingly, and in the most water-efficient way.
- Install a compost bin for your food scraps and garden waste. Compost is good for your garden and reduces the amount of waste going to landfill.
- To help support wildlife, choose plants that attract bees and other pollinators. Consider building an insect hotel. Insects are important in gardens: as well as pollinating plants, they also eat pests and attract other wildlife into the garden, such as birds.
- Use more environmentally friendly ways to control weeds and pests – for example, choose organic weed killers, mulch the soil, encourage predator insects.

WHAT CAN WE DO AT WORK?

Check if there is an environmental policy or sustainability committee. If there is, many of the following ideas should be in place. If not, you can still do your bit and encourage others to do the same. For instance:

- Reduce, reuse and recycle, just as you would at home.
- Use environmentally friendly paper, only print when necessary, print on both sides of the paper and alter the ink setting (print as draft).
- Turn off electronics (don't leave on stand by), lighting and heating before you go home.
- Recycle toner and ink cartridges.
- Walk or cycle to work, or use public transport. If a car is necessary, try to car-share with a colleague to reduce the amount of fossil fuel being used.

FOOD, DRINK AND SHOPPING

Avoid Disposable Plastic

- Avoid buying bottled water.
- Use a refillable water bottle and take it everywhere you go, filling up from a tap where possible. Many places like shopping centres, airports, shops, cafés, hotels and restaurants are now providing water stations for refilling bottles. Look online or download a mobile app to help you find your nearest refilling station, or look out for a window sticker which lets you know that they are participating in a "free water" refill scheme.
- Don't use a plastic straw. If required, use an alternative such as paper, glass, bamboo or metal.
- Avoid using disposable cutlery.
- Carry a reusable coffee cup for drinks on the move. Many coffee shops now offer an incentive for people who bring their own cup.
- Use your own shopping bags rather than plastic bags supplied by shops.
- Don't buy products containing microbeads. Many countries have now banned microbeads in cosmetics and personal care products but they may still be found in some countries, so check the labels.
- It is possible to "refill" many products (such as coffee or handwash) so check a product for this option.

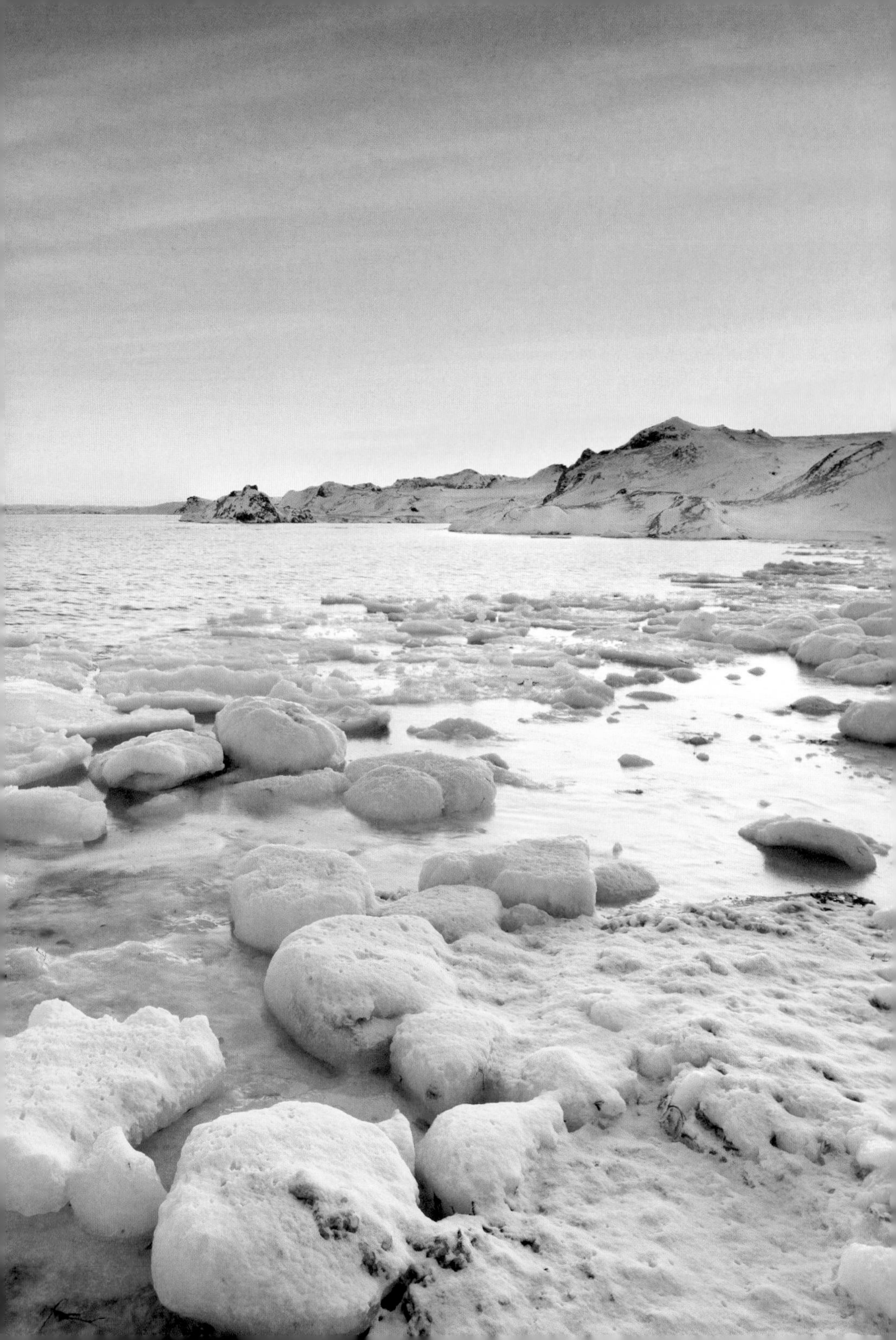

Buy Sustainable Seafood

- Consult a consumer guide for information on the species that are the most – and least – sustainable. There are guides available for many countries. The World Wide Fund for Nature website has a list[179].
- Look for certification labels on seafood packaging in supermarkets. These labels indicate that a fishery has been through an assessment process and its catch is currently deemed sustainable.
- Look online for a list of sustainable seafood restaurants in your area. Some restaurants are extremely active in the support and promotion of sustainable seafood but, if no information is available, ask restaurant staff about the sources of the seafood on their menu.
- Support initiatives and campaigns that encourage sustainable seafood use.

WHAT CAN WE DO ON HOLIDAY?

If you can, consider a staycation – fewer flights are better for the environment. If you do go away, try to be a sustainable traveller. Some people book ecotourism holidays which aim to minimize the impact tourism has on fragile and beautiful environments and their local communities, but you can always find ways to reduce your impact on the environment, whether at home or abroad. For instance, you can:

- Carbon offset your flight.
- Bag and bin your litter or take it home.
- Reduce your waste while away (use your own shopping bags, use a refillable water bottle, and so on).
- Reduce water and energy use (many countries have limited supplies of both).
- Research "wildlife experiences" carefully before booking.
- Buy locally (food, accommodation, souvenirs), especially products that may help the environment or the communities you visit (see page 175).
- Don't buy products made from endangered species such as sea turtles, or marine curios such as shells, dried seahorses or coral. Although not all species for sale may currently be illegal or rare, supporting the curio trade encourages exploitation of species and damage to habitats during collection.
- Eat ethically: when trying local exotic foods, do not eat rare or endangered species (such as shark's fin soup or Bluefin tuna). Try to eat sustainable species.
- As the saying goes, "Take only pictures, leave only footprints".

The Problem with Lionfish

Lionfish (*Pterois* spp) are beautiful but venomous marine fish that are native to the waters of the Indo-Pacific. Two species, however, have invaded the east coast of the United States and the Caribbean – and are spreading down the east coast of South America. It is unknown exactly how lionfish became an invasive species – possibly through accidental or deliberate release from aquaria – but they are now a major threat to the ecology of the coral reefs, mangroves and seagrass beds they invade. Their voracious appetites, lack of predators, and high rates of reproduction and growth dramatically reduce the abundance and diversity of native fish. As it is currently impossible to eradicate the lionfish, the best that can be achieved is some level of control.

Communities are becoming increasingly inventive in the ways to tackle their local lionfish problem – and you can help too. Lionfish are good to eat, so try them if you see them on the menu. Some communities organize "Lionfish Derbies" – a competition where teams try to remove as many lionfish as they can in one day. Prizes are awarded to winning teams, and there are filleting and cooking demonstrations for the public to watch. Buying lionfish jewellery is another way you could help. Not only does the buying of lionfish jewellery incentivize lionfish removal by adding value to lionfish catches, but it provides an additional form of welcome income for local households.

WHAT CAN WE DO AT THE BEACH OR ON THE COAST?

- If on a kayak or out in a boat, don't throw anything overboard.
- Take all your litter home.
- Always pick up after your dog and make sure it doesn't foul beaches (or anywhere else).
- Avoid disturbing wildlife on the beach or in the water, including sea birds, dolphins, basking sharks and seals (use binoculars for a better view of marine life).
- **Dolphins**: boats should stay a minimum of 100m (110yds) away. If dolphins actively approach your boat, switch the engine to neutral. Do not pursue the dolphins if they move away. Avoid groups of dolphins with mothers and young. Use boat skippers who adopt these practices, checking social media for recommendations.
- **Basking sharks**: boats should stay at least 100m (110yds) away (see page 177).
- **Seals**: keep 100m (110yds) from seals out of the water. Do not walk through a group of seals, especially mothers nursing pups. If a seal moves into the water, it can indicate that the seal has been disturbed – rushing into the sea causes the seal physical damage and may scare other seals. Move slowly away; you are already too close. If in a boat, keep quiet and do not rev boat engines. If you see a seal in the water, slow to less than 5 knots and remain parallel to the seal to avoid disturbing it – and always allow it an escape route. If a seal approaches your boat maintain your course at a slow speed or stop. Don't forget, you can always use binoculars for a better view!
- There are many organizations that would be interested in your sightings of these marine species – look online to see who to contact.
- Report dead or injured animals to the appropriate organization.

Basking Sharks

The following guidelines help boat handlers reduce the risk of killing, injuring or harassing basking sharks.

- Restrict your speed to below 6 knots and avoid sudden speed changes.
- When closer than 100m (110yds), switch the engine to neutral to avoid injuring sharks.
- Avoid disturbing dense groups of sharks as you may disrupt courtship behaviour.
- Be extremely cautious in areas where basking sharks have been seen breaching.
- Remember that for every shark visible on the surface, there are likely to be more hidden just below.
- Take time to observe the direction of movement of the basking sharks to anticipate their course – you can then position yourself for the best view.
- If you have a camera with you, take a picture of the dorsal fin – photographs may contribute valuable data to a photo-identification project.
- Jet-skis are incompatible with basking sharks and should stay at least 500m (550yds) away.

The Rock Pool Code

- Respect seashore creatures.
- Do not splash in the rock pool. You are likely to see more animals if you are still and quiet.
- Try not to cast a shadow over the pool as this will startle the animals and make them hide away.
- Gently push aside seaweed and carefully lift up rocks to look for rock pool creatures. Leave animals where you find them – do not pull them out of crevices or try to prise them off rocks. Return the rocks to the position you found them in.
- If you wish to see the animal more closely, gently catch it with a net – or preferably your hands – so as not to damage it, then pop it in a bucket. Only look at one animal at a time – keeping several in a bucket at once may stress them.

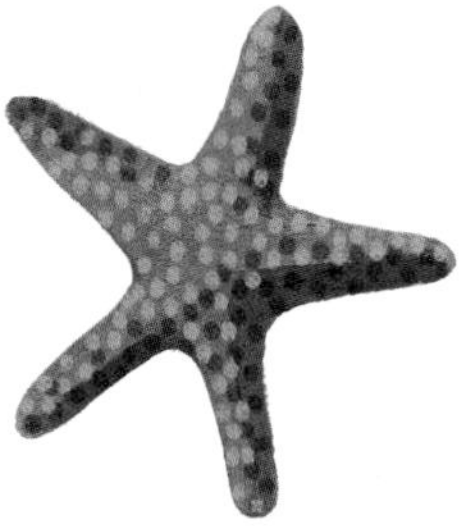

- Do not keep the creature in the bucket for long as the oxygen in the water will run low – return the animal carefully to the pool as soon as possible.
- Rock-pooling is best done at low tide but take care to keep an eye on the tide so that you don't get into difficulties.

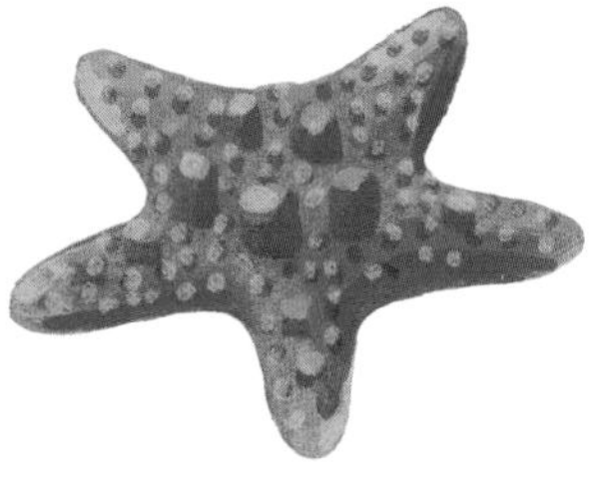

- Advise young children of this best practice for viewing rock pools with minimum environmental impact.

BUYING PRODUCTS FOR THE BEACH

Think about the products you buy for the beach. More and more sustainable products are now available.

- Surfboards – a greater range of more environmentally friendly materials are now available for surfboards. More surfboards are being made using materials that are sustainably sourced (for example wooden boards), or use renewable, recycled and/or upcycled materials. Materials and processes that reduce toxicity during the manufacturing process are also being used more frequently now. Look for boards displaying the Level One or the Gold Level ECOBOARD logo.[180]

- Swimwear can now be made from regenerated nylon (ECONYL®) obtained from landfill and the oceans.

- Some innovative projects, such as Net-Works™ [181], are working with coastal communities to encourage the recovery of discarded nylon fishing nets from their local seas. Collected nets are made into environmentally friendly carpet tiles. These initiatives help clean up littered beaches and villages, reduce "ghost fishing" (whereby discarded nets trap and injure marine life), and provide communities with valuable income.

- Other products produced from recycled fishing nets include:
  – Accessories such as sunglasses, bracelets, necklaces.
  – Clothing and footwear such as socks, outdoor gear.
  – Homeware and garden accessories such as mats and rugs.
  – Recreation products such as skateboards, fishing equipment and frisbees.

How to Improve Your Pro-environmental Credentials

- Help with a beach clean – and encourage others to do the same.
- Become more "ocean literate" – learn more about the marine environment and wildlife in your area and what you can do to help.
- Sign a petition or write to your local authority about an issue you feel passionately about.
- Support charities and organizations that care for the oceans, either financially or by volunteering your time.
- If you Tweet, follow #OceanOptimism, a Twitter initiative established in 2014 to spread the word about marine conservation success stories.
- Join a "Citizen Science" project and help collect or analyse data for the scientific community. There are several projects focusing on the marine and coastal environment that you may be able to help locally or online. Here are some projects currently available:

  – **The Great Eggcase Hunt Project**: aims to get as many people as possible to hunt for and record shark, skate and ray eggcases which have either been washed ashore, or are found by divers and snorkelers underwater.
  – **Basking Shark Project**: contribute your sightings to the database.
  – **Off the Hook**: anglers are encouraged to record their catch records.
  – **Shark Sightings Database**: contribute your sightings to the database.
  – **Whale track**: if living or visiting Scotland, download the Hebridean Whale and Dolphin Trust mobile app and report your sightings.

– **Floating Forests**: an online project which helps scientists identify past and present kelp forests from an enormous number of satellite images.
– **iSeahorse**: a project to identify and map seahorses for conservation.
– **Seagrass Spotter**: everyone from fishers to scuba divers can contribute to a global project to map seagrass meadows to help protect them.
– **Plankton Portal**: this online project helps scientists classify plankton from a huge number of images at sea.
– **Marine Invaders**: a project inviting people to spend 10 minutes surveying one of three types of marine site (such as rocky shore) to check for and log non-native (invasive) species. There is a similar project based in Australia.
– **Surfing for Science**: this project has been monitoring the coastal environment with the help of surfers who have temperature sensors and GPS attached to their surfboards. There is potential to expand this project to include other watersports users.

The Future of Blue Health Research

One of the most positive and exciting steps towards the protection of our oceans is the increasing realization of the indirect, non-material benefits of the marine environment to human health and well-being. While the value of the marine environment for climate regulation, food, fuel, pharmeceuticals, and so on is well-known, it is only relatively recently that greater attention is being directed towards the less obvious benefits – emotional, social, cultural and spiritual. Some new avenues of research are particularly innovative:

- **Virtual and Augmented Reality**: Studies involving virtual and augmented reality technology may be important in helping future healthcare professionals to provide alternative ways that the elderly, or those with limited mobility, can experience the restorative benefits of the seas.
- **Biodiversity**: As we have seen, the impact of biodiversity on health and wellbeing may extend far beyond the availability of species we can exploit: we increasingly appreciate how the presence of flora and fauna can impact how we feel. While research to date has tended to focus on the positive benefits of viewing biodiversity, it stands to reason that, conversely, we may suffer negative effects if biodiversity is lost. In view of this, further research will continue to explore our complex relationship with the nature around us, for the benefit of all.
- **WEIRD sampling**: The overwhelming majority of scientific research carried out has used people from Western, Educated, Industrialized, Rich, and Democratic countries ("WEIRD"), despite the fact that most of the world's population lives in developing countries. Important steps, however, are now being made to research the relationships that people from less developed countries have with their seas and coasts. This is imperative if, collectively, in both developed and developing countries, we intend in the future to repair and take care of our oceans.

In the words of Dr Sylvia Earle, renowned marine biologist, oceanographer and explorer, "We need to respect the oceans and take care of them as if our lives depended on it. Because they do."

REFERENCES

1 https://www.oceanicinstitute.org/aboutoceans/aquafacts.html

2 United Nations (n.d.) Percentage of total population living in coastal areas. Retrieved from http://www.un.org/esa/sustdev/natlinfo/indicators/methodology_sheets/oceans_seas_coasts/pop_coastal_areas.pdf on 23 May 2018

3 Wheeler, B. W., White. M., Stahl-Timmins, W. & Depledge, M. H. (2012). Does living by the coast improve health and wellbeing? *Health and Place*, 18, 1198–1201

4 Hattam, C., Beaumont, N. & Austen, M. (2014). The seas, ecosystem services, and human wellbeing. In Bowen, R. E., Depledge, M. H., Carlarne, C. P. & Fleming, L. E. (Eds). *Oceans and Human Health: Implications for Society and Wellbeing*. (pp. 71–112). John Wiley & Sons, Ltd

5 MacNaughton, R. B., Cole, J. M., Dalrymple, R. W., Braddy, S. J., Briggs, D. E. G. & Lukie, T. D. (2002). First steps on land: Arthropod trackways in Cambrian-Ordovician eolian sandstone, southeastern Ontario, Canada. *Geology*, 30, 391–394

6 Ashbullby, K. J., Pahl, S., Webley, P. & White, M. P. (2013). The beach as a setting for families' health promotion: a qualitative study with parents and children living in coastal regions in Southwest England. *Health and Place*, 23, 138–147

7 Wheeler, B., White, M. P., Fleming, L. E., Taylor, T., Harvey, A., & Depledge, M. H. (2014). Influences of the oceans on human health and wellbeing. In Bowen., R. E., Depledge, M. H., Carlarne, C. P. & Fleming, L. E. (Eds). *Oceans and Human Health: Implications for Society and Wellbeing*. (Cpt. 1; pp. 3–22). John Wiley & Sons, Ltd, Chichester, UK

8 WHO (World Health Organization) (1946). Preamble to the Constitution of the World Health Organization as adopted by the International Health Conference, New York, 19–22 June, 1946; signed on 22 July 1946 by the representatives of 61 States (*Official Records of the World Health Organization*, no. 2, p. 100) and entered into force on 7 April 1948. Geneva: WHO

9 Bell, S. L., Phoenix, C., Lovell, R. & Wheeler, B. W. (2015). Seeking everyday wellbeing: The coast as a therapeutic landscape. *Social Science & Medicine*, 142, 56–67

10 WHO (2013). Mental health action plan 2013–2020. Retrieved from http://www.who.int/mental_health/publications/action_plan/en/ on 18 December 2015

11 Dodge, R., Daly, A. P., Huyton, J. & Sanders, L. D. (2012). The challenge of defining wellbeing. *International Journal of Wellbeing*, 2, 222–235

12 Ulrich, R. S., Simons, R. F., Losito, B. D., Fiorito, E., Miles, M. A. & Zelson, M. (1991). Stress recovery during exposure to natural and urban environments. *Journal of Environmental Psychology*, 11, 201–230

13 Wallace, R. A., Sanders, G. P. & Ferl, R. J. (1991). *Biology: the Science of Life*. New York: HarperCollins Publishers Inc. (pp. 899–902).

14 HSE (2017). Health and safety at work summary statistics for Great Britain 2017, Retrieved from http://www.hse.gov.uk/Statistics/overall/hssh1617.pdf on 22 May 2018

15 European Agency for Safety and Health at Work – EU-OSHA (2014). European Risk Observatory (Calculating the cost of work-related stress and psychosocial risks) European Risk Observatory Literature Review

16 WHO (2017). World Mental Health Day 2017 – Mental health in the workplace. Retrieved from http://www.who.int/mental_health/world-mental-health-day/2017/en/ on 22 May 2018

17 Health Council of the Netherlands and Dutch Advisory Council for Research on Spatial Planning, Nature and the Environment. Nature and Health. The influence of nature on social psychological and physical wellbeing. The Hague: Health Council of the Netherlands and RMNO, 2004: publication no. 2004/09E; RMNO publication nr A02ae

18 Bowler, D. E., Buyung-Ali, L. E., Knight, T. M. & Pullin, A. S. (2010). A systematic review of evidence for the added benefits to health of exposure to natural environments. *BMC Public Health*, 10, 456

19 Velarde, M. D., Fry, G. & Tveit, M. (2007). Health effects of viewing landscapes – landscape types in environmental psychology. *Urban Forestry & Urban Greening*, 6, 199–212

20 Hughes, J., Pretty, J. & Macdonald, D. W. (2013). Nature as a source of health and wellbeing: is this an ecosystem service that could pay for conserving biodiversity? In Macdonald, D. W. & Willis, K. J. (Eds.) *Key Topics in Conservation Biology 2* (pp. 143–160). Chichester, West Sussex, UK: Wiley-Blackwell

21 Hartig, T. (2004). Toward understanding the restorative environment as a health resource. Open space–People space: An international conference on inclusive environments. Retrieved from http://www.openspace.eca.ac.uk/conference/proceedings/PDF/Hartig.pdf on 16 January 2014

22 Hartig, T., Mitchell, R., De Vries, S. & Frumkin, H. (2014). Nature and health. *Annual Review of Public Health*, 35, 21.1–21.22

23 Miller, J. R. (2005). Biodiversity conservation and the extinction of experience. *TRENDS in Ecology and Evolution*, 20: 430–434

24 St Leger, L. (2003). Health and nature – new challenges for health promotion. *Health Promotion International*, 18, 173–175

25 Ulrich, R. S. (1983). Aesthetic and affective response to natural environment. In Altman, I. and Wohwill, J. F. (Eds.). *Behaviour and the Natural Environment* (pp. 85–125). New York: Plenum

26 Ulrich, R. S. (1984). View through a window may influence recovery from surgery. *Science*, 224, 420–421

27 Ulrich, R. S. (1993). Biophilia, biophobia and natural landscapes. In Kellert, S. & Wilson, E. O. (Eds.). *The Biophilia Hypothesis* (pp. 73–137). Washington DC: Island Press

28 Hartig, T., Evans, G. W., Jamner, L. D., David, D. S. & Gärling, T. (2003). Tracking restoration in natural and urban field settings. *Journal of Environmental Psychology*, 23, 109–123

29 Berto, R. (2005). Exposure to restorative environments helps restore attentional capacity. *Journal of Environmental Psychology*, 25, 249–259

30 Pretty, J., Peacock, J., Sellens, M. & Griffin, M. (2005). The mental and physical outcomes of green exercise. *International Journal of Environmental Health Research*, 15, 319–337

31 Laumann, K., Gärling, T. & Stormark, K. M., (2001). Rating scale measures of restorative components of environments, *Journal of Environmental Psychology*, 21, 31–44.

32 Laumann, K., Gärling, T. & Stormark, K. M., (2003). Selective attention and heart rate responses to natural and urban environments. *Journal of Environmental Psychology*, 23, 125–134

33 Kweon, B. S., Ulrich, R. S., Walker, V. D. & Tassinary, L. G. (2008). Anger and stress: the role of landscape posters in an office setting. *Environment and Behavior*, 40, 355–381

34 Nanda, U., Eisen, S. L. & Baladandayuthapani, V. (2008). Undertaking an art survey to compare patient versus student art preferences. *Environment and Behavior*, 40, 269–301

35 Schneider, S. M. & Hood, L. E. (2007). Virtual reality: A distraction intervention for chemotherapy. *Oncology Nursing Forum*, 34, 39–46

36 Tanja-Dijkstra K., Pahl S., White M. P., Andrade J., Qian C., Bruce M. & Moles, D. R. (2014). Improving dental experiences by using virtual reality distraction: A Simulation Study. *PLoS ONE*, 9: e91276. Doi:10.1371/journal.pone.0091276

37 Huang, S. C. L. (2009). The validity of visual surrogates for representing waterscapes. *Landscape Research*, 34, 323–335

38 Hull, R. B. & Stewart, W. P. (1992). Validity of photo-based scenic beauty judgements. *Journal of Environmental Psychology*, 12, 101–114

39 Kjellgren, A. & Buhrkall, H. (2010). A comparison of the restorative effect of a natural environment with that of a simulated natural environment. *Journal of Environmental Psychology*, 30, 464–474

40 Mayer, F. S., Frantz, C. M., Bruehlman-Senecal, E. & Dolliver, K. (2009). Why is nature beneficial?: The role of connectedness to nature. *Environment and Behavior*, 41, 607–643

41 Shafer, E. L. & Richards, T. A. (1974). A comparison of viewer reactions to outdoor scenes and photographs of those scenes. USDA Forest Service Research Paper NE-302

42 McMahan, E. A. & Estes, D. (2015). The effect of contact with natural environments on positive and negative affect: A meta-analysis. *The Journal of Positive Psychology*, doi:10.1080/17439760.2014.994224

43 Bratman, G. N., Hamilton, J. P. & Daily, G. C. (2012). The impacts of nature experience on human cognitive function and mental health. *Annals of the New York Academy of Sciences*, 1249, 118–136

44 Gascon, M., Triguero-Mas, M., Martinez, D., Dadvand, P., Forns, J., Plasència, A. & Nieuwenhuijsen, M. J. (2015). Mental health benefits of long-term exposure to residential green and blue spaces: A systematic review. *International Journal of Environmental Research and Public Health*, 12, 4354–4379

45 Luttik, J. (2000). The value of trees, water and open space as reflected by house prices in the Netherlands. *Landscape and Urban Planning*, 48, 161–167

46 Lange, E., & Schaeffer, P. V. (2001). A comment on the market value of a room with a view. *Landscape and Urban Planning*, 55, 113–120

47 White, M., Pahl, S., Wheeler, B. W., Fleming, L. E. F. & Depledge, M. H. (2016). The 'Blue Gym': What can blue space do for you and what can you do for blue space? *Journal of the Marine Biological Association*, 96, 5–12

48 Coss, R. G., Ruff, S. & Simms, T. (2003). All that glistens: II. The effects of reflective surface finishes on the mouthing activity of infants and toddlers, *Ecological Psychology*, 15, 197–213

49 White, M., Smith, A., Humphryes, K., Pahl, S., Snelling, D. & Depledge, M. (2010). Blue space: The importance of water for preference, affect, and restorativeness ratings of natural and built scenes. *Journal of Environmental Psychology*, 30, 482–493

50 Berman, M. G., Jonides, J. & Kaplan, S. (2008). The cognitive benefits of interacting with nature. *Psychological Science*, 19, 1207–1211

51 Herzog, T. R. (1985). A cognitive analysis of preferences for waterscapes, *Journal of Environmental Psychology*, 5, 225–241

52 Simaika, J. P. & Samways, M. J. (2010). Biophilia as a universal ethic for conserving biodiversity. *Conservation Biology*, 24, 903–906

53 Heerwagen, J. (2009). Biophilia, health, and wellbeing. In: Campbell, L. & Wiesen, A. (Eds). *Restorative commons: creating health and wellbeing through urban landscapes.* (pp. 38–57). Gen. Tech Rep. NRS-P-39. U.S. Department of Agriculture, Forest Service, Northern Research Station;

54 Wilson, E. O. (1993). Biophilia and the conservation ethic. In Kellert, S. & Wilson, E. O. (Eds.). *The Biophilia Hypothesis* (pp. 31–41). Washington DC: Island Press

55 Kellert, S. R. (2008). Biophilia. In Jørgensen, S. E. & Fath, B. D. (Eds.). *Encyclopedia of Ecology* (pp. 462– 466). Amsterdam, Netherlands: Elsevier

56 van den Berg, M. M. H. E., Maas, J., Muller, R., Braun, A., Kaandorp, W., van Lien, R., van Poppel, M. N. M., van Mechelen, W. & van den Berg, A. E. (2015). Autonomic Nervous System Responses to Viewing Green and Built Settings: Differentiating Between Sympathetic and Parasympathetic Activity. *International Journal of Environmental Research and Public Health*, 12, 15860–15874

57 Kaplan, R. & Kaplan, S. (1989). *The Experience of Nature: A Psychological Perspective*. New York, U.S., Cambridge University Press

58 Kaplan, S., Bardwell, L. V. & Slakter, D. B. (1993). The museum as a restorative environment. *Environment and Behavior*, 25, 725–742

59 Kaplan, S. (1995). The restorative benefits of nature: toward an integrative framework. *Journal of Environmental Psychology*, 15, 169–182

60 Pol, E. (2006). Blueprints for a History of Environmental Psychology (I): From First Birth to American Transition. *Medio Ambiente y Comportamiento Humano*, 7, 95–113

61 Gifford, R. (2014). Environmental psychology matters. *Annual Review of Psychology*, 65, 541–79

62 Domingo, J. L. (2007). Omega-3 fatty acids and the benefits of fish consumption: Is all that glitters gold? *Environment International*, 33, 993–998

63 Cornish, M. L. & Garbary, D. J. (2010). Antioxidants from macroalgae: potential applications in human health and nutrition, *Algae*, 25, 155–171

64 Rajapakse, N. & Kim, S-K. (2011). Chapter 2 Nutritional and digestive health benefits of seaweed *Advances in Food and Nutrition Research*, 64, 17–28

65 Anjum K., Abbas, S. Q., Shah, S. A. A., Akhter, N., Batool, S. & ul Hannan, S. S. (2016). Marine sponges as a drug treasure. *Biomolecules and Therapeutics*, 24, 347–362

66 Charlier, R. H. & Chaineux, M-C. P. (2009). The Healing Sea: A Sustainable Coastal Ocean Resource: Thalassotherapy. *Journal of Coastal Research*, 25, 838–856

67 Fenical, W. (1996). Marine biodiversity and the medicine cabinet – The status of new drugs from marine organisms. *Oceanography* 9, 23–27

68 FAO website. Antimicrobial resistance – What you need to know. Retrieved from http://www.fao.org/zhc/detail-events/en/c/451065/ on 11 June 2018

69 WHO website. Antibiotic resistence. Retrieved from http://www.who.int/news-room/fact-sheets/detail/antibiotic-resistance on 11 June 2018

70 Bell, S., Lovell, R., Hollenbeck, J., White, M. & Depledge, M. (2018). Coastal health: risks and benefits. In Foley, R., Kearns, R., Kistemann, T. & Wheeler, B. (Eds). *Blue Space, Health and Wellbeing: Hydrophilia Unbounded* (Chp. 9); Oxford, Routledge.

71 Ernst, E. (2000). The role of complementary and alternative medicine. *British Medical Journal*, 321, 1133–1135

72 Gröber, U., Werner, T., Vormann, J. & Kister, K. (2017). Myth or Reality—Transdermal Magnesium? *Nutrients*, 9, 813; doi:10.3390/nu9080813

73 Watkins, K. & Josling, P. D. (2010) A Pilot Study to determine the impact of Transdermal Magnesium treatment on serum levels and whole body CaMg Ratios. *European Journal for Nutraceutical Research*, pp. 8

74 NHS website. Benefits of exercise. Retrieved from https://www.nhs.uk/live-well/exercise/exercise-health-benefits/ on 4 Jun 2018

75 Elkins, M. R., Robinson, M., Rose, B. R., Harbour, C., Moriarty, C. P., Marks, G. B….& Bye, P. T. P. (2006). A Controlled Trial of Long-Term Inhaled Hypertonic Saline in Patients with Cystic Fibrosis. *New England Journal of Medicine*, 354, 229–24

76 Barton J. & Pretty J. (2010). What is the best dose of nature and green exercise for improving mental health? A multi-study analysis. *Environmental Science and Technology*, 44, pp. 3947–3955

77 Focht, B. C. (2009). Brief walks in outdoor and laboratory environments: effects on affective responses, enjoyment, and intentions to walk for exercise. *Research Quarterly for Exercise and Sport*, 80, pp. 611–620

78 Ceci R. & Hassmen P. (1991). Self-monitored exercise at three different RPE intensities in treadmill vs field running. *Medicine and Science in Sports and Exercise*, 23, pp. 732–738

79 Bird, W. (2007). Natural Thinking. Investigating the links between the Natural Environment, Biodiversity and Mental Health. A report for the Royal Society for the Protection of Birds (pp. 116)

80 Depledge, M. H. & Bird, W. J. (2009). The Blue Gym: Health and wellbeing from our coasts. *Marine Pollution Bulletin*, 58, 947–948.

81 Young, N. (1983). *The History of Surfing – Nat Young with Craig McGregor and Rod Holmes*. Palm Beach Press (pp. 224)

82 Elliott, L. R., White, M. P., Grellier, J., Rees, S. E., Waters, R. D. & Fleming, L. E. (2018). Recreational visits to marine and coastal environments in England: Where, what, who, why, and when? *Marine Policy*, https://doi.org/10.1016/j.marpol.2018.03.013

83 White, M. P., Wheeler, B. W., Herbert, S., Alcock, I. & Depledge, M. H. (2014). Coastal proximity and physical activity: is the coast an under-appreciated public health resource? *Preventative Medicine*, 69, 1350140

84 Lee, I-M. & Buchner, D. M. (2008). The Importance of Walking to Public Health. *Medicine and Science in Sports and Exercise*, 40, pp. S512–S518

85 Elliott, L. R., White, M. P., Grellier, J., Rees, S. E., Waters, R. D. & Fleming, L. E. (2018). Recreational visits to marine and coastal environments in England: Where, what, who, why, and when? *Marine Policy*, https://doi.org/10.1016/j.marpol.2018.03.013

86 White, M. P., Bell, S., Elliott, L., Jenkin, R., Wheeler, B. W. & Depledge, M. H. (2016). The health effects of blue exercise in the UK. In Barton, J., Bragg, R., Wood, C. & Pretty, J. (Eds), *Green Exercise: Linking Nature, Health and Wellbeing* (Chp 7, pp. 69–78); Oxford, Routledge

87 Takeshima, N., Rogers, M. E., Watanabe, E., Brechue, W. F., Okada, A., Yamada, T., Islam, M. M. & Hayano, J. (2002). Water-based exercise improves health-related aspects of fitness in older women. *Medicine and Science in Sports and Exercise*, 34, 544–51

88 de Andrade, S. C., de Carvalho, R. F., Soares, A. S., de Abreu Freitas, R. P., de Medeiros Guerra, L. M. & Vilar, M. J. (2008). Thalassotherapy for fibromyalgia: a randomized controlled trial comparing aquatic exercises in sea water and water pool. *Rheumatology International*, 29, 147–152

89 Learning Outside the Classroom website: http://www.lotc.org.uk/

90 Hignett, A., White, M. P., Pahl, S., Jenkin, R. & Le Froy, M. (2018). Evaluation of a surfing programme designed to increase personal wellbeing and connectedness to the natural environment among 'at risk' young people. *Journal of Adventure Education and Outdoor Learning*, 18, 53–69

91 Nichols, W. J. (2014). Red mind, grey mind, blue mind: The health benefits of water. In *Blue Mind: How water makes you happier, more connected and better at what you do* (pp. 139–181). Little, Brown and Company, United States

92 Telford, R. M., Telford, R. D., Olive, L. S., Cochrane, T. & Davey, R. (2016). Why are girls less physically active than boys? Findings from the LOOK longitudinal study. *PLoS ONE*, 11(3), e0150041. doi:10.1371/journal.pone.0150041

93 Craft, B. B., Haley A., Carroll, H. A. & Lustyk, M. K. B. (2014). Gender Differences in Exercise Habits and Quality of Life Reports: Assessing the Moderating Effects of Reasons for Exercise. *International Journal of Liberal Arts and Social Science*, 2(5): 65–76

94 Poulain, M., Pes, G. M., Grasland, C., Carru, C., Ferruccid, L., Baggio, G., Franceschi, C. & Deiana, L. (2004). Identification of a geographic area characterized by extreme longevity in the Sardinia island: the AKEA study, *Experimental Gerontology*, 39, 1423–1429

95 Global Wellness Summit (2018). 2018 Wellness Trends, from Global Wellness Summit Report Copyright © 2017–2018 by Global Wellness Summit. Retrieved from https://www.globalwellnesssummit.com/2018-global-wellness-trends/ on 10 April 2018

96 Healthline website: https://www.healthline.com/nutrition/10-reasons-why-good-sleep-is-important#section10 on 4 June 2018

97 Ratcliffe, E. (2015). Sleep, mood and coastal walking. Report prepared for The National Trust. Retrieved from https://www.nationaltrust.org.uk/documents/sleep-mood-and-coastal-walking---a-report-by-eleanor-ratcliffe.pdf on 3 June 2018

98 Daniels, S. L. (2002). On the ionization of air for removal of noxious effluvia (Air ionization of indoor environments for control of volatile and particulate contaminants with nonthermal plasmas generated by dielectric-barrier discharge). IEEE Transactions on Plasma Science, 30, 1471–1481

99 Perez, V., Alexander, D. D. & Bailey, W. H. (2013). Air ions and mood outcomes: a review and meta-analysis. *BMC Psychiatry*, 13, 29

100 NHS website. Retrieved from https://www.nhs.uk/conditions/vitamins-and-minerals/vitamin-d/ on 4 June 2018

101 Bahrami, A., Mazloum, S. R., Maghsoudi, S., Soleimani, D., Khayyatzadeh, S. S., Arekhi, S. … & Ghayour-Mobarhan, M. (2017). High Dose Vitamin D Supplementation Is Associated With a Reduction in Depression Score Among Adolescent Girls: A Nine-Week Follow-Up Study, *Journal of Dietary Supplements*, 15, 173–182

102 Vidgren, M., Virtanen, J. K., Tolmumen, T., Nurmi, T., Tuomainen, T.-P., Voutilainen, S. & Ruusunen, A. (2018). Serum Concentrations of 25-Hydroxyvitamin D and Depression in a General Middle-Aged to Elderly Population in Finland. *The Journal of Nutrition, Health and Aging*, 22, 159–164

103 Williams, C. E., Williams, E. A. & Corfe, B. M. (2018). Vitamin D status in irritable bowel syndrome and the impact of supplementation on symptoms: what do we know and what do we need to know? *European Journal of Clinical Nutrition*, doi: 10.1038/s41430-017-0064-z

104 Aranow, C. (2011). Vitamin D and the immune system. *Journal of Investigative Medicine*, 59, 881–886

105 NHS website. Retrieved from https://www.nhs.uk/conditions/metabolic-syndrome/ on 4 June 2018

106 Schmitt, E. B., Nahas-Neto, J., Bueloni-Dias, F., Poloni, P. F., Orsatta, C. L. & Nahas, E. A. P. (2018). Vitamin D deficiency is associated with metabolic syndrome in postmenopausal women. *Maturitas*, 107, 97–102

107 Ali, M. N. & Vaidya, V. (2007). Vitamin D and cancer, *Journal of Cancer Research and Therapeutics*, 3, 225–230

108 Giovannucci, E., Liu, Y., Rimm, E. B., Hollis, B. W., Fuchs, C. S., Stampfer, M. J. & Willett, J. C. (2006). Prospective Study of Predictors of Vitamin D Status and Cancer Incidence and Mortality in Men. *Journal of the National Cancer Institute*, 98, 451–459

109 Volker, S. & Kistemann, T. (2011). The impact of blue space on human health and wellbeing – Salutogenic health effects of inland surface waters: A review. *International Journal of Hygiene and Environmental Health*, 214, 449–460

110 Yamashita, S. (2003). Perception and evaluation of water in landscape: use of photo-projective method to compare child and adult residents' perceptions of a Japanese river environment. Landscape and Urban Planning, 62, 3–17.

111 Korpela, K. M., Hartig, T., Kaiser, F. G. & Fuhrer, U. (2001). Restorative experience and self-regulation in favorite places. *Environment & Behavior*, 33, 572–589

112 White, M. P., Pahl, S., Ashbullby, K., Herbert, S. & Depledge, M. H. (2013). Feelings of restoration from recent nature visits. *Journal of Environmental Psychology*, 35, 40–51

113 Pearson, D. G. and Craig, T. (2014). The great outdoors? Exploring the mental health benefits of natural environments. *Frontiers in Psychology*, 5, 1178. Doi: 10.3389/fpsyg.2014.01178

114 Mitchell, R. & Popham, F. (2008). Greenspace, urbanity and health: relationships in England. *Journal of Epidemiology and Community*, 61, 681–683

115 Peng, C., Yamashita, K. & Kobayashi, E. (2016). Effects of the coastal environment on wellbeing. *Journal of Coastal Zone Management*, 19, DOI: 10.4172/2473-3350.1000421

116 Palmer, S. E. & Schloss, K. B. (2010). An ecological valence theory of human color preference. *Proceedings of National Academy of Science*, 107, 8877–8882

117 Nichols, W. J. (2014). The senses, the body, and "Big Blue". In *Blue Mind: How water makes you happier, more connected and better at what you do* (pp. 79–104). Little, Brown and Company, United States

118 BBC website: Retrieved from http://www.bbc.co.uk/homes/design/colour_psychologyofcolour.shtml#blue_ on 18 June 2018

119 Today website: https://today.yougov.com/topics/international/articles-reports/2015/05/12/why-blue-worlds-favorite-color on 18 June 2018

120 White, M. P., Cracknell, D., Corcoran, A., Jenkinson, G. & Depledge, M. H, (2014). Do preferences for waterscapes persist in inclement weather and extend to sub-aquatic scenes? *Landscape Research*, 39, 339–358

121 Hägerhäll, C. M., Laike, T., Küller, M., Marcheschi, E., Boydston, C. & Taylor, R. P. (2015). Human Physiological Benefits of Viewing Nature: EEG Responses to Exact and Statistical

Fractal Patterns. *Nonlinear Dynamics, Psychology, and Life Sciences*, 19, 1–12.

122 Gillis, K. & Gatersleben, B. (2015). A Review of Psychological Literature on the Health and Wellbeing Benefits of Biophilic Design. Buildings, 5, 948–963.

123 Pérez-Martínez, G., Torija, A. J. & Ruiz, D. P. (2018). Soundscape assessment of a monumental place: A methodology based on the perception of dominant sounds. *Landscape and Urban Planning*, 169, 12–21

124 Rew, K. (2008). *Wild Swim: River, Lake, Lido And Sea: The Best Places To Swim Outdoors In Britain*. London: Guardian Books

125 Kjellgren, A. & Westman, J. (2014). Beneficial effects of treatment with sensory isolation in flotation-tank as a preventive health-care intervention – a randomized controlled pilot trial. *BMC Complementary & Alternative Medicine*, 14, 417

126 White, M. P., Weeks, A., Hooper, T., Bleakley, L., Cracknell, D., Lovell, R. & Jefferson, R. L. (2017). Marine wildlife as an important component of coastal visits: The role of perceived biodiversity and species behaviour. *Marine Policy*, 78, 80–89

127 Cracknell, D., White, M. P., Pahl, S., Nichols, W. J. & Depledge, M. H. (2016). Marine biota and psychological wellbeing: A preliminary examination of dose–response effects in an aquarium setting. *Environment and Behavior*, 48, 1242–1269. DOI: 10.1177/0013916515597512

128 Jefferson, R. L., Bailey, I., Laffoley, D. d'A., Richards, J. P. & Attrill, M. J. (2014). Public perceptions of the UK marine environment. *Marine Policy*, 43, 327–337

129 Kellert, S. R. (1993). The biological basis for human values of nature. In Kellert, S. & Wilson, E. O. (Eds.). *The Biophilia Hypothesis* (pp. 42–69). Washington DC: Island Press

130 Woods, B. (2000). Beauty and the Beast: Preferences for animals in Australia. *The Journal of Tourism Studies*, 11, 25–35

131 Cracknell, D., White, M. P., Pahl, S. & Depledge, M. H. (2017). A preliminary investigation into the restorative potential of public aquaria exhibits: A UK student-based study. *Landscape Research*, 42, 18–32

132 Lindemann-Matthies, P., Junge, X. & Matthies, D. (2010). The influence of plant diversity on people's perception and aesthetic appreciation of grassland vegetation. *Biological Conservation*, 143, 195–202

133 Curtin, S. (2009). Wildlife tourism: the intangible, psychological benefits of human–wildlife encounters. Current Issues in Tourism, 12, 451–474.

134 Cziksentmihalyi, M. (1990). *Flow – The Psychology Of Optimal Experience*. New York: Harper & Row

135 Marino, L. & Lilienfeld, S. O. (2007). Dolphin-Assisted Therapy: More Flawed Data and More Flawed Conclusions. *Anthrozoös*, 20, 239–249

136 Nimer, J. & Lundahl, B. (2007). Animal-assisted therapy: A meta-analysis. *Anthrozoös*, 20, 225–238

137 Wortman, R. A., Vallone, T., Karnes, M., Walawander, C., Daly, D. & Fox-Garrity, B. (2018). Pinnipeds and PTSD: An Analysis of a Human-Animal Interaction Case Study Program for a Veteran. *Occupational Therapy International*, Vol 2018, Article ID 2686728, https://doi.org/10.1155/2018/2686728

138 Kidd, A. H. & Kidd, R. M. (1999). Benefits, problems, and characteristics of home aquarium owners. *Psychological Reports*, 84, 998–1004

139 Ginsburg, K. R. and the Committee on Communications and the Committee on Psychosocial Aspects of Child and Family Health (2007). The Importance of Play in Promoting Healthy Child Development and Maintaining Strong Parent-Child Bonds. *Pediatrics*, 119, 182–191

140 Hipp, J. A. & Ogunseiten, O. A. (2011). Effect of environmental conditions on perceived psychological restorativeness of coastal parks. *Journal of Environmental Psychology*, 31, 421–429

141 Wyles, K. J., Pahl, S., Thomas, K. & Thompson, R. C. (2016). Factors That Can Undermine the Psychological Benefits of Coastal Environments: Exploring the Effect of Tidal State, Presence, and Type of Litter. *Environment and Behavior*, 48, 1095–1126

142 Grellier J., White M. P., Albin, M., Bell, S., Elliott, L. R., Gascón, M. … & Fleming, L. E (2017). BlueHealth: a study programme protocol for mapping and quantifying the potential benefits to public health and wellbeing from Europe's blue spaces. *BMJ Open* 2017;7:e016188. doi:10.1136/bmjopen-2017-016188

143 Casagrande website: Retrieved from https://www.casagrandelaboratory.com/marco-casagrande/ on 3 July 2018

144 Thompson Coon, J., Boddy, K., Stein, K., Whear, R., Barton, J., & Depledge, M. H. (2011). *Environmental Science and Technology*, 45, 1761–1772

145 Caddick, N., Smith, B. & Phoenix, C. (2015). The Effects of Surfing and the Natural Environment on the WellBeing of Combat Veterans, *Qualitative Health Research*, 25, 76–86

146 Virtual Reality Society website: retrieved from https://www.vrs.org.uk/virtual-reality/what-is-virtual-reality.html on 29 June 2018

147 Stone, R. J., Small, C., Knight, J. F., Qian, C. & Shingari, V. (2014). Virtual Environments for Healthcare Restoration and Rehabilitation. Invited Chapter (Part VI) in Ma, M., Jain, L. C. & Anderson, P. (Eds.) *Virtual and Augmented Reality in Healthcare 1*. Intelligent Systems Reference Library 68; Springer-Verlag: Heidelberg, Germany; pp. 497–521

148 Tanja-Dijkstra, K., Pahl, S., White, M. P., Auvray, M., Stone, R. J., Andrade, J., May, J., Mills, I. & Moles, D. R. (2017). The Soothing Sea: A Virtual Coastal Walk Can Reduce Experienced and Recollected Pain. *Environment & Behavior*, 1–27 DOI: 10.1177/0013916517710077

149 BlueHealth Project website: https://bluehealth2020.eu/ on 18 June 2018

150 White, M. P., Smith, A., Humphries, K., Pahl, S., Snelling, D. & Depledge, M. H. (2010). Blue Space: The importance of water for preference, affect and restorative ratings of natural and built scenes. *Journal of Environmental Psychology*, 30,482–493

151 Gould van Praag, C. D. (2017). Mind-wandering and alterations to default mode network connectivity when listening to naturalistic versus artificial sounds. *Scientific Reports*, 7, 45273

152 Ali, B., Al-Wabel, N. A., Shams, S., Ahamad, A., Khan, S. A. & Anwar, F. (2015). Essential oils used in aromatherapy: A systemic review. *Asian Pacific Journal of Tropical Biomedicine*, 8, 601–611

153 Van Dierendonck, D. & Te Nijenhuis, J. (2005). Flotation restricted environmental stimulation therapy (REST) as a stress-management tool: A meta-analysis, *Psychology and Health*, 20, 405–412

154 Murck H. (2002). Magnesium and affective disorders, Nutritional Neuroscience, 5, 375–89

155 Abbasi, B., Kimiagar, M., Sadeghniiat, K., Shirazi. M. M., Hedayati, M. & Rashidkhani B., (2012). Journal of Research in Medical Sciences, 17, 1161–9

156 Morgan P., Salacinski A. & Stults-Kolehmainen M., (2013). The Journal of Strength and Conditioning Research, 27, 3467–74

157 Vartanian, O. & Suedfeld, P. (2011). The Effect of the Flotation Version of Restricted Environmental Stimulation Technique (REST) on Jazz Improvisation, *Music and Medicine*, doi:10.1177/1943862111407640

158 Pimentel, F. B., Alves, R. C., Rodrigues, F. & Oliveira, M., (2017). Macroalgae-Derived Ingredients for Cosmetic Industry—An Update, *Cosmetics*, 5, 2

159 Thomas, N. V. & Kim, S-K., (2013). Beneficial Effects of Marine Algal Compounds in Cosmeceuticals. *Marine Drugs*, 11, 146–64

160 Choi, J-S., Bae, H-J., Kim, S-J. & Choi, I. S. (2011). In vitro antibacterial and anti-inflammatory properties of seaweed extracts against acne inducing bacteria, Propionibacterium acnes. *Journal of Environmental Biology*, 32, 313–18

161 Shibata, T., Fujimoto, K., Nagayama, K., Yamaguchi, K. & Nakamura, T. (2002). Inhibitory Activity Of Brown Algal Phlorotannins Against Hyaluronidase. *International Journal of Food Science and Technology*, 37, 703–9

162 Yamori, Y., Miura, A. & Taira, K (2001). Implications From And For Food Cultures For Cardiovascular Diseases: Japanese Food, Particularly Okinawan Diets. Asia Pacific Journal of Clinical Nutrition, 10, 144–5

163 Atashrazm, F., Lowenthal, R. M., Woods, G. M., Holloway, A. F. & Dickinson, J. L. (2015). Fucoidan and Cancer: A Multifunctional Molecule with Anti-Tumor Potential. Marine Drugs, 13, 2327–2346

164 Fitzgerald, C., Gallagher, E., Tasdemir, D. & Hayes, M. (2011). Heart Health Peptides from Macroalgae and Their Potential Use in Functional Foods. *Journal of Agricultural and Food Chemistry*, 59, 6829–6836

165 Woodroffe, C. D., Nicholls, R. J., Burkett, V. & Forbes, D. L. (2014). The impact of climate change of coastal ecosystems. In Bowen., R. E., Depledge, M. H., Carlarne, C. P. & Fleming, L. E. (Eds). *Oceans and Human Health: Implications for Society and Wellbeing* (Cpt 6, pp. 141–176). John Wiley & Sons, Ltd, Chichester, UK

166 Jezkova, T. & Wiens, J. J. (2016). Rates of change in climatic niches in plant and animal populations are much slower than projected climate change. Proceedings of the Royal Society B, 283: 20162104. http://dx.doi.org/10.1098/rspb.2016.2104

167 Queiroz, N., Humphries, N. E., Mucientes, G., Hammerschlag, N., Lima, F. P., Scales, K. L., Miller, P. I., Sousa, L. L., Seabra, R. & Sims, D. W. (2016). Ocean-wide tracking of pelagic sharks reveals extent of overlap with longline fishing hotspots. *Proceedings of the National Academy of Sciences U.S.A.*, 113, 1582–1587

168 Naylor, R. L., Goldburg, R. J., Primavera, J., Kautsky, N., Beveridge, M. C. M., Clay, J., Folke, C., Lubchenco, J., Mooney, H. & Troell, M. (2001). Effects of Aquaculture on World Fish Supplies. *Issues in Ecology*, 8, 1–8

169 Goksøyr, A. (2006). Endocrine Disruptors in the Marine Environment: Mechanisms of Toxicity and their Influence on Reproductive Processes in Fish. *Journal of Toxicology and Environmental Health*, Part A, 69, 175–184

170 Wilson, M. I., Robertson, L. D., Daly, M. & Walton, S. A. (1995). Effects of visual cues on assessment of water quality. *Journal of Environmental Psychology*, 15, 53–63

171 Kamrowski, R. L., Limpus, C., Moloney, J. & Hamann, M. (2012). Coastal light pollution and marine turtles: assessing the magnitude of the problem. Endangered Species Research, 19, 85–98.

172 Salmon, M. (2003). Artificial night lighting and sea turtles. *Biologist*, 50, 163–168

173 Weilgart, L. S. (2007). The impacts of anthropogenic ocean noise on cetaceans and implications for management. *Canadian Journal of Zoology*, 85, 1091–1116

174 Gall, S. C. & Thompson, R. C. (2015). The impact of debris on marine life. *Marine Pollution Bulletin*, 92, 170–179

175 Van Cauwenberghe, L. & Janssen, C. R. (2014). Microplastics in bivalves cultured for human consumption. *Environmental Pollution*, 193, 65–70

176 Smith, N. (2018). Where did all the sand go? *Engineering and Technology (E&T Magazine)*, Vol. 13, issue 7/8 (August/September), 22–25

177 Desprez, M. (2000). Physical and biological impact of marine aggregate extraction along the French coast of the Eastern English Channel: short and long-term post-dredging restoration. *ICES Journal of Marine Science*, 57, 1428–1438

178 Spurling, A. (2018). Where did all the sand go? *Engineering and Technology (E&T Magazine)*, Vol. 13, issue 7/8 (August/September), 46–49

179 http://wwf.panda.org/get_involved/live_green/out_shopping/seafood_guides/

180 http://www.sustainablesurf.org/ecoboard/

181 http://net-works.com/

INDEX

PICTURE CREDITS

Alamy Stock Photo JHeinimann 41.

Getty Images Ippei Naoi 70–1; Jethuynh 128–9.

iStock armiblue 144–5; barbaraaaa 143; borchee 83; cinoby 52–3; DarrenTierney 22–3; den-belitsky 64–5; dtokar 131; franckreporter 123; IBorisoff 78; johnandersonphoto 164–5; kn1 75; kokkai 47; lubilub 88–9; Maica 72–3; naumoid 44; nonimatge 167; pixelfit 12–13; Rike_ 68–9; sara_winter 172; Sergey Lisitsyn 120–1; shaunl 170–1; turner890 138; USO 34.

Jenny McConnell Front cover artwork.

Pixabay Free-Photos 93.

Unsplash Adam Bixby 160–1; Afrah 15; Ammar Elamir 86–7; Arno Smit 37; Austin Neill 48–9; Erik Jan Leusink 97; Ian Schneider 4–5; Iswanto Arif 81; Jamie Street 180–1; Jason Briscoe 26–7; Jorg Angeli 32–3; Kees Streefkerk 25; Kilarov Zaneit 8; Michael Olsen 124; Noah Usry 30; Rosan Harmens 98; Rube Gutierrez 110; Samule Sun 148; Sean O 60–1; Shawn Ang 154; Shifaaz Shamoon 18; Sora Sagano 118.

ACKNOWLEDGEMENTS

I would like to thank for Kate Adams for approaching me about writing this book, and for her contributions on pages 9–10.

I would like to thank Jo Smith for her contributions on pages 92–115, 119 and 122–51.

Thank you to Jo Smith and Leanne Bryan for editorial assistance.

I've enjoyed working with you all.

Thank you to Professor Michael Depledge, who started me on this research path, and also to Drs Mathew White and Sabine Pahl, for their encouragement in taking on this venture.

Special thanks to Malcolm Woodward, who read my first drafts and subsequent frequent changes. Thank you, Malc – you've been a huge help and support.